Couples, Conflict, and Change

Social work with marital relationships

Adrian L. James and
Kate Wilson

TAVISTOCK PUBLICATIONS
London and New York

To our families

First published in 1986 by
Tavistock Publications Ltd
11 New Fetter Lane, London EC4P 4EE

© 1986 Adrian L. James and Kate Wilson

Phototypeset by Boldface Typesetters, London
Printed in Great Britain by
Richard Clay (The Chaucer Press) Ltd
Bungay, Suffolk

British Library Cataloguing in Publication Data

James, Adrian L.
   Couples, conflict, and change: social work
   with marital relationships. – (Tavistock library
   of social work practice)
   1.   Family social work – Great Britain
   I.   Title   II. Wilson, Kate
   362.8'253   HV700.G7

ISBN 0-422-79900-9
ISBN 0-422-79910-6 Pbk

Contents

General editor's foreword

Historically, social work theory paid close attention to marital problems, and a good deal of scarce resources were devoted to marital counselling by a number of the pre-Seebohm specialist agencies. Since Seebohm this theoretical and practice commitment has waned under the weight of the reorganization of the personal social services, the expansion of the statutory responsibilities, and the ever-increasing demand for services. It is now clear that this hasty abandonment was ill-judged, and the realization that the cause of many of our clients' miseries is rooted in their most intimate marital and sexual relationships has been revived. So far, however, this revival has not resulted in publications which consider not only the nature of problems facing couples in conflict, but also the particular contribution which social workers might make to their resolution. Further, standard works tend to interpret marital problems within a rather narrow psychodynamic perspective, and to concentrate on marriage and marital breakdown, rather than on an understanding which considers marriage and family life within the wide and complex array of social, economic, interpersonal, and sexual factors which influence it, or in terms of the particular approaches which social workers might adopt to promote solutions.

This book remedies this situation by closely examining the problems facing couples in conflict in terms of the dramatic social, legal, and sexual changes which have occurred since the last war; the nature of marital problems; the roles and tasks of the social worker attempting to contribute to the resolution of these difficulties; the different approaches to marital therapy which the social worker might adopt. It also discusses 'conciliation' as an approach which is uniquely suited to working with problems arising out of marital difficulties. In

addition the book provides a succinct summary of the legal framework relating to marriage and marital breakdown.

The authors of this volume – currently lecturers in the Department
of Social Administration at Hull University – have experience in probation and in working with family and marital problems, and also
work as voluntary conciliators with a probation service. They have
collaborated in research and other publications, and each has published independently.

This book is one of a series in the Tavistock Library of Social Work
Practice, designed to represent the collaborative effort of social work
academics, practitioners, and managers. In addition to considering
the theoretical and philosophical debate surrounding the topics
under consideration, the texts are firmly rooted in practice issues and
the problems associated with the organization of the services. Therefore the series will be of particular value to undergraduate and postgraduate students of social work and social administration.

The Tavistock Library of Social Work Practice series was prompted
by the growth and increasing importance of the social services in our
society. Until recently there has been a general approbation of social
work, reflected in a benedictory increase in manpower and resources,
which has led to an unprecedented expansion of the personal social
services, a proliferation of the statutory duties placed upon them, and
major reorganization. The result has been the emergence of a profession faced with the immense responsibility of promoting individual
and social betterment, and bearing a primary responsibility to advocate on behalf of individuals and groups who do not always fulfil or
respect normal social expectations of behaviour. In spite of the
growth in services these tasks are often carried out with inadequate
resources, an uncertain knowledge base, and as yet unresolved difficulties associated with the reorganization of the personal social services in 1970. In recent years these difficulties have been compounded
by a level of criticism unprecedented since that attracted by the Poor
Law. The anti social work critique has fostered some improbable alli-
ances between groups of social administrators, sociologists, doctors,
and the media, united in their belief that social work has failed in its
general obligation to 'provide services to the people', and in its particular duty to socialize the delinquent, restrain parents who abuse their
children, prevent old people from dying alone, and provide a satisfactory level of community care for the sick, the chronically handicapped,
and the mentally disabled.

These developments highlight three major issues that deserve particular attention: first, the need to construct a methodology for analysing social and personal situations and prescribing action; second, the necessity to apply techniques that measure the performance of the individual worker and the profession as a whole in meeting stated objectives; third, and outstanding, the requirement to develop a knowledge base against which the needs of clients are understood and decisions about their care are taken. Overall, the volumes in this series make explicit and clarify these issues; contribute to the search for the distinctive knowledge base of social work; increase our understanding of the aetiology and care of personal, familial, and social problems; describe and explore new techniques and practice skills; aim to raise our commitment towards low status groups which suffer public, political, and professional neglect; and promote the enactment of comprehensive and socially just policies. Above all, these volumes aim to promote an understanding which interprets the needs of individuals, groups, and communities in terms of the synthesis between inner needs and the social realities that impinge upon them, and which aspire to develop informed and skilled practice.

M. Rolf Olsen, 1986

Acknowledgements

In the process of writing this book we have received help, support, and encouragement from many friends and colleagues. Particular thanks must go to Dorothy Whitaker and Douglas Hooper for their advice on various problems, and to Martin Parry, who kindly read the Appendix on the law. Thanks must also go to Gilbert Smith and Robert Chester for their interest and encouragement, and also to the latter for his permission to quote from unpublished material, and to Rolf Olsen for his editorial assistance.

We also owe a large debt to past clients and students, and to many practitioners for additional case material and comment. In particular, our thanks to Rani Atma of the NMGC Asian Counselling Project in Bradford, Brian Cantwell of the Humberside Probation Service, John Corden of the Leeds FSU, Bridget Atkinson and a small group of social workers from Humberside Social Services who met with us to share their experiences.

Thanks must also go to the several secretarial colleagues who helped at various stages in the drafting process, particularly Tricia Daly, Pat Moody, and Margaret White. Finally, we owe a very special debt to our respective spouses for their support and encouragement throughout.

Preface

Social workers and probation officers cannot help but be aware of the fundamental importance of marriage and similar intimate pair relationships to their clients and their families, not only as a source of strength, support, and satisfaction, but also as the springhead of many of their frustrations, trials, and tribulations. Yet evidence from a wide range of sources indicates that social-work intervention in such relationships is much less frequent than might be expected. The reasons for this, some of which we discuss in this book, are manifold, but an important factor in our view is that intervention in such problems is seen by many social workers to require arcane knowledge and esoteric skills. This view has been reinforced substantially by the relatively limited amount that has been written in Britain about this area of practice, frequently from what might be regarded as highly specialized points of view, which seem to bear little relationship to the practice world of most social workers in either voluntary or statutory agencies.

Our purpose in this book therefore is to try to remedy this situation by providing social workers, when faced with possible marital problems, with ideas as to how they might understand and conceptualize these and set about offering help. We have summarized a wide range of material relating to marriage, some of which may already be familiar to students and practitioners, but which has not until now been brought together in readily accessible form. Where space has prevented a full discussion, we have indicated sources and further reading, so that the book will serve as a useful reference point as well as a textbook.

Part I places marital problems in an historical, societal, and theoretical context, considering both a wide range of problems and problem-generating situations, and a range of theoretical approaches to understanding these. Part II offers a discussion of a range of approaches to intervention that are substantially derived from but not necessarily dependent upon these, with which many social workers will be already familiar. By discussing marital problems in the context of familiar practice frameworks, we have attempted to show how social workers can, in working with marital problems, draw upon the knowledge and skills that they already possess.

In the process of taking a more eclectic approach, we have sought to follow 'mainstream' social-work thinking and have therefore been unable to incorporate many of the richly diverse approaches that can be found in social-work theory and practice today. But it is our hope that, as a result, our attempt at demystification will encourage many social workers to feel more confident about their skills and therefore more ready to engage in this area of work.

We have tended to use the term 'marital' to describe all couples who are in intimate pair relationships, whether they are legally married or not. To have qualified this on each occasion would have been pedantic. Similarly, we have used the terms 'pairs', 'couples', 'partners', and 'dyads' interchangeably. Our concern throughout, however, regardless of terminology, is with the individuals involved in the 'marital' relationship.

PART I

Understanding marital problems

1
The state of marriage

The family, marriage, and the individual are inextricably inter-woven. This simple fact constitutes a major conceptual and practical problem when considering the prospect of intervention in a marital problem, for it militates against clarity of thought and purpose. Certainly, conceptual distinctions can be made, and these are of central importance in the attempts of social scientists to shed light on the dynamics of family life; but such distinctions tend to rely upon the identification of boundaries that are perhaps seldom recognized, let alone drawn, by the individual experiencing the realities of marital and family life. As the father of modern family studies, William J. Goode (1964), observed, 'We know too much about the family to be able to study it both objectively and easily' (Goode 1964:3).

This is perhaps the very core of the problem, for every one of us 'knows', from our unique personal experiences, about marriage and family life. Now, more than at any time in Britain's history, marriage is an almost universal phenomenon, as is the raising of a family for those who do marry. Almost all of us spend our formative years in a family; even though in 1978 there were over 100,000 children in the care of local authorities, this was less than 1 per cent of the relevant age group, and a substantial minority of these were in foster homes. Furthermore, 60 per cent of children admitted into care leave within eight weeks (Study Commission on the Family 1980:39). Thus the experience of family life for children is virtually universal. Even those who do not marry will have been profoundly influenced by their parents' marriage, their experience of which as children may even be part of the reason for their remaining unmarried. There will also be those, who are also the subject of this book, who forego the religious and civil formalities of marriage, but none the less enter into an intimate couple relationship with all the other characteristics of marriage. For them, and for those who do marry, the marriages of their respective parents will exert a powerful influence on their expectations, perceptions, and behaviour in their own marriages, until long after the start of their relationship.

It would therefore be a fruitless task to draw contentious distinctions between marriage and the family, although it is clear they are not synonymous. Our concern in this book, however, is primarily with the marital relationship, but recognizing that this is influenced by factors both in the immediate family environment and in the wider social environment.

It is of central importance to locate the marital relationship and the family, both of which are currently the focus of much debate and anxiety amongst the institutions of the state and amongst the general public, in an historical framework. The importance of this initial task for our examination of social work with marital problems lies in the fact that many current expressions of concern about marriage and the family seem to hinge upon the notion of a 'golden age' of family life in times past, which has become a powerful force in our perception of and attitudes towards the family and marriage today, a thesis recently explored by Pearson (1983) in relation to delinquency. Underlying much of the current concern is the fact that the family unit, centred on the marital dyad, is regarded by many as the institution that is the corner-stone of society. As the Rapoports have argued,

> 'Families . . . have been our most durable social unit. From hunting and gathering bands through the most complex modern State, family units have been adapting to, and at the same time influencing, the course of development of other parts of society.'
>
> (Rapoport and Rapoport 1982:475)

They suggest that British families today are in a state of transition from coping with a society that had a single overriding norm of family life, to one in which a plurality of norms are seen as legitimate and may even be desirable.

From the central importance of the family, other commentators have helped to develop the mythology of a 'golden age'. For example, Dicks (1967) has described the traditional family in glowing terms as a three- or four-generational group that provided a rich and meaningful environment for its members, in contrast to the modern urban family, which he characterizes as its 'vestigial' and 'shrunken' successor. He suggests

that many of the difficulties in modern marriages are the result of
rapid change in family structure and a failure to adapt to new realities
of family life. Gathorne-Hardy refers to the belief in a stable golden
era in the past, conjuring up images of 'a calm, traditional, settled
community where marriages, too, were settled and enduring'
(1981:28). Kay has argued that

> 'The characteristics of Western marriage were for generation after
> generation based on permanent monogamy, a patriarchal head,
> and insistence that junior members shall obey and respect the
> seniors. All these traits . . . are now being challenged by the family
> itself.'   (1972:9)

Rapoport and Rapoport (1982) have also argued that there is evidence of an almost universal decline in the authority that elders have
in organizing the marital and family life of their children; of widespread changes in the rights and obligations of the 'extended' network
of kin and community ties; and evidence of a widespread decline in
the size of domestic groups.

Perhaps the 'model family' most commonly referred to in the current debate is that of the nuclear family composed of legally married
couples, voluntarily choosing the parenthood of one or two children,
all of who reside together as a distinct domestic unit. In fact, however,
only about 4 in 10 of all British households conform to this model, and
A. Oakley has argued that 'Judged by statistical criteria alone, the
conventional family is no longer "normal". On the contrary, it is not,
at any given time, the prevailing social arrangement' (1982:125). Yet
this model remains a powerful influence in the minds of many, as does
the traditional extended family with its many supposed virtues. The
reality of such views and models will shortly be explored, but the significance of the mythology of marriage and family life, which is largely
independent of fact, is that it provides the major source of the ideals
that we express in debate and attempt to embody in our own marital
and family relationships. It is therefore also frequently the source of
much of our anguish, frustration, and disappointment. In an attempt
to put this mythology into perspective, therefore, we must examine
the changes that have taken place within the family and its environment and the implication of these for individuals within the family,
and particularly for those at its core, the marital dyad.

6 Couples, conflict, and change

The history of marriage and the family

An historical analysis of marriage and the family is important in the current climate of concern because 'Even quite general knowledge about the past can have a calming effect. It is the only way to acquire perspective, to find out what is important and what is not' (Gathorne-Hardy 1981:27). The undertaking of such an historical analysis by non-historians is a task fraught with difficulties, not least of which is the critical evaluation of differing accounts and reconstructions. Such a task is made more difficult by developments within the discipline that have led some historians to talk of a rejection of traditional historical preoccupations with the reconstruction of particular events and more recent attempts 'to seek understanding at another and even more elusive level' (Rosenberg 1975:2). This involves seeking an appreciation of the emotional texture of life for individuals in the past, their feelings, their perceptions, and the factors that influenced their choices, both social and moral, through the use of a wide range of qualitative data – literature, letters, diaries, journals, sermons, etc. – which are frequently under-used by social historians, perhaps because such materials pose problems of interpretation. And yet the attempt must be made because these are precisely the issues that are likely to tell us most about the way marital and family life was experienced in the past and help us to determine the extent to which the proposed existence of an earlier 'golden age' is myth or reality.

The starting point for such an analysis is to some extent arbitrary and dictated by expediency in the sense that few records survive from the first centuries of English history. Gathorne-Hardy has suggested from the available evidence, however, that

> 'it is likely that up to the eleventh century divorce was easy, and casual sleeping around and affairs were common . . . . This reveals not immorality so much as a completely different sexual and marital morality – one which to a certain extent echoes some developments today. Marriage was not expected to last for life.' (1981:16)

In similar vein, Mount has concluded that 'The most regular and universal feature of non-Christian or pre-Christian marriage is the relative ease of divorce' (1982:200); throughout a great deal of recorded history, marriage has been primarily a private contract that could be ended in the same way it was entered into, by mutual consent given either in writing or before witnesses.

As the Church increased its power, this right to divorce was gradually eroded as it sought to establish control over and to regulate the estate of marriage, its purpose being, according to Mount, 'to minimise the uncleanness of sexual intercourse, to regulate sex for those who could not aspire to the superior state of celibacy' (1982:202). This process was not complete until about 1300, but from that time the system of divorce derived from canon law prevailed virtually unchanged until the twentieth century. A major consequence of this was that the Church, with its substantial control over the written word, was largely able to blanket the resentment of the unhappily married, presenting thereby a somewhat distorted picture for historians to interpret.

Family structure

It is against this background that the evidence relating to the nature of the family and family life, and its impact upon the marital relationship, needs to be considered. The belief in the existence of a traditional extended family model is shared by some historians. Laslett talks of 'a very general supposition that in the past the domestic group was universally and necessarily larger and more complex than it is today in industrial cultures' (1972a:5). He goes on to describe this as a 'belief or misbelief [that] certainly seems to display a notable capacity to overlook contrary facts and to resist attempts at revision' (1972a:8).

This belief arose partly because historians and sociologists throughout Western Europe have ignored the importance of the developmental cycle of the family – starting and often ending with the married couple living on their own, with the inevitable changes in size and composition during the child-rearing years – and of demographic issues. Goody was led to conclude that 'it is not only for England that we need to abandon the myth of the extended family' (1972:124). Laslett (1972a) has concluded that the mean household size of 4.75 persons, including 2.73 children, has remained relatively constant from the sixteenth century to the beginning of the present century. The size of the domestic group did not begin to fall sharply until 1891, which can be attributed almost entirely to the fall in the number of servants especially after 1911, since when it has continued to fall. There were some variations, especially between social classes, with a tendency at the upper levels of society for larger households, which was a result of the inclusion of servants in the figures for household composition. In general, however, 'very few households can be identified containing more than two generations – parents and their children' (Laslett 1972b:152).

The impact of the Industrial Revolution on marital and family life must also be considered. Before the rise of capitalism, husband, wife, and children formed the unit of economic production; labour was divided within families by age and by sex; and the roles of both sexes were equally valued. The worlds of marriage, the family, and work were one and the same. With the growth of factory production, these previously integrated elements were separated so that a division occurred between work and personal life that led to women being assigned new and specialized roles as primary carers, at a time when economic circumstances and prevailing social values facilitated the close identification of women with the home. Indeed, the Victorian era saw the evolution of these beliefs in such a way that they came to be seen almost as a moral imperative. At the same time, Oakley (1982) argues, these beliefs did not match with the realities of women's daily lives, neither in working-class nor in middle-class contexts; in fact, they constituted what amounts to a mythology. This was none the less a powerful and pervasive mythology with which was associated a whole constellation of values and attitudes relating to marriage and family life, which still influences ideas of how the family should behave and has been evident in much of the recent debate about social policy and family life (Segal 1983).

The evidence suggests that this separation of family and work, and its contribution to the emergence of a powerful ideology of women's roles and family life, was not totally without foundation. For example, most women operating in the Lancashire cotton mills in the mid-nineteenth century were under twenty-one, and only 25 per cent were married (Scott and Tilly 1975). There is also evidence from other cotton towns that households with children under ten where the wife worked were three times as likely to include a residing grandmother, and that paradoxically in some industrial areas the effect of industrialization was the *growth* of extended family households:

> 'It seems likely that urban–industrial life of the cotton-town type markedly increased the proportion of wage earner families in which parents and married children co-resided. It also markedly increased the alternative form of residence for the young married couple, living as lodgers with another family.'(Anderson 1972:225)

Similarly, few old people lived apart from a relative. In some towns over 80 per cent of old people were living with one of their children, a substantially higher proportion than can be found today, although the situation was worse in rural areas. Anderson also observes that 'it was possible for employed children to continue to live at home until they married . . . . By contrast, in the country, though the relationships with their parents of those who did remain at home were almost certainly closer, only a bare majority were able to remain at home until they married.'   (1972:233)

Many had to migrate to towns or leave home for economic reasons, to become a domestic or farm servant in the household of another family.

The overall impact of the Industrial Revolution on family life was thus not as massive or even as negative as is commonly supposed. Whilst it caused fundamental changes by separating home and work, with substantial consequences for marital and family life, the increased earnings of both husbands and working wives made it possible for them to keep their parents, who could then look after the grandchildren. This has led Mount (1982) to observe that, contrary to conventional wisdom, only since the Industrial Revolution, and then mainly in industrial towns, have married couples started to live with their parents in three-generational households in any great numbers. In so far as it exists at all, therefore, the extended family is a modern development. 'Despite its barbarities and deprivations, one thing that the Industrial Revolution did *not* do was break up families' (Mount 1982:55).

Marital and family relationships

The discussion has so far focussed primarily on the structure of the family in history, because this provides the framework within which most marriages exist. In addition, some historians have recently attempted to provide an interpretation of the 'emotional texture' of married and family life and how this was affected by broader social, economic, and political changes. There is a tendency, evident in much of the debate about the climbing divorce rates, to infer that marriage used to be more stable and more enduring, even allowing for more restrictive divorce laws. But as Stone (1977) points out, the age of the first marriage was very late for the majority in sixteenth-century England, except for male heirs and daughters of families in the landed classes. Even in early-nineteenth-century England, nearly 30 per cent of all marriages were broken by death in the first fifteen years:

'the duration of marriage was generally very short . . . if one adopts the reasonable criterion of durability, marriages in the mid-twentieth century were more stable than at almost any other time in history, despite the high divorce rate.'   (Stone 1977:55)

Thus, Stone suggests, modern divorce is little more than a functional substitute for death, which society was forced to adopt as an institutional escape-hatch from broken marriages with the decline in the adult mortality rate after the late eighteenth century.

Once again, a different picture begins to emerge. Married couples had a less than 50 per cent statistical probability of continued life together for more than a couple of years after their children had left home; and remarriage was therefore very common, with about 25 per cent of all marriages being a remarriage for either the bride or the groom. The result was that 'in the seventeenth century the remarriage rate, made possible by death, was not far off that in our own day, made possible by divorce' (Stone 1977:56).

Marriages by widows and widowers with stepchildren of their own, or families that included orphaned or even abandoned nieces or nephews, were comparatively common, with perhaps a quarter of all families being hybrid or reconstituted families of this sort. There was also a high infant and child mortality rate of between 30 and 50 per cent affecting all classes, although the poor suffered more than the rich; this rate did not begin to fall until the late eighteenth century, and less than half of the children who survived into adulthood did so while both their parents were alive. Thus only a small minority of parents lived long enough to become an economic burden on their children in their old age. Stone concludes that, in statistical terms, pre-modern marital and family relationships were temporary and transient:

'the omnipresence of death coloured affective relations at all levels of society, by reducing the amount of emotional capital available for prudent investment in any single individual, especially in such ephemeral creatures as infants.'   (Stone 1977:651−52)

This resulted in

'a conjugal family which was very short-lived and unstable in its composition. Few mutual demands were made on its members, so that it was a low-keyed and undemanding institution which could therefore weather this instability with relative ease.'(Stone 1977:60)

Shorter (1976) echoes Stone, claiming that good mothering is essentially an invention of modern society, in which the welfare of the child is paramount. In traditional society, because of the high infant and child mortality rates, the development and happiness of children − especially those under the age of two − were viewed with indifference by the mother. Mount dismisses this as 'the strangest myth of all' (1982:104), arguing that the evidence suggests that the huge number of abandoned children was related to poverty rather than to inherent lack of caring by parents. Furthermore, family practices such as sending children away into domestic service or as hired labour to another farm – both common in pre-industrial England, continuing well into the nineteenth century and even into the early twentieth century (see, for example, Kitchen 1942) – were a reflection of predominant economic pressures rather than affectionless families (Mount 1982). As these divisive economic pressures relaxed, so families were better able to stay together, whereas in the past they had clung together as best they could:

'To deduce from the sad fragments of evidence which came down to us from this harsh world that men and women had no feelings for one another or for their children is the most callous act of historical condescension.'   (Mount 1982:130)

Mount suggests that, even as far back as the beginning of the thirteenth century, 'love within marriage, fully articulated, passionate sexual love, was a familiar and admired phenomenon in the nobility' (1982:62), and that in the sixteenth century, the earliest period for which there is reliable evidence, arranged marriages were the exception rather than the rule. It was only amongst the nobility and the landed classes that the laws of primogeniture retained much significance and marriages of convenience were the rule; as late as 1537 young couples still had the power, in spite of the efforts of the Church to regulate marriage, to marry themselves simply by exchange of vows. This power sprang from the principle of Christian canon law that true marriage depended upon freely given consent and therefore could not be separated from affection – which, Mount argues, is evident in the records of the ecclesiastical courts.

Although divorce was legally difficult to obtain, marriages did break down, the consequences of which in the sixteenth and seventeenth centuries, for a wife with children and no family to take her in, could be severe. Records suggest that children and deserted wives formed a large proportion of the poor. Mount concludes that none of the direct evidence fits in with Stone's view of marriage; on the contrary,

'the emotional intensity of the relationship and the risks of failure leave an unmistakable impression. Marriage was a central experience in the life of every human being and the end of a marriage – whether caused by death or desertion – was likely to prove a desolating event.'   (1982:87)

Although some marriages were underpinned by economic or political motivations, Mount suggests that these factors could not have wholly determined what happened after the marriage. The very fact of living together in the same household inevitably creates emotional connections, and although many marriages were short-lived, between 1500 and 1800 one-fifth of all marriages lasted thirty-five years or more, which compares favourably with marriages today. Mount also suggests that, whilst a feminist critique of marriage and the family argues that women were expected, indeed compelled, to assume secondary roles, to be passive, unassertive, modest, and directed towards marriage and the pleasure and service of men, this may be only part of the picture, since there is evidence throughout history of hen-pecked husbands and assertive women. Mount also dismisses as another myth the notion that women in the past were mostly unacquainted with sexual pleasure, a view that does not stand up to historical examination once the 'official propaganda of polite society in the high Victorian age' (1982:223) has been placed in its proper social and historical context. If, as the evidence suggests, women were not only experiencing sexual pleasure but in fact demanding it and complaining when it was not forthcoming, then women could not have been as unequal in the most personal and intimate aspects of marriage as we are commonly led to believe.

This is not to suggest that some women, or even many, were not oppressed to varying degrees — but merely to strive for perspective and a balanced view. The commonly supposed legal inequality of women appears to have applied primarily, and even then not entirely, to the laws of inheritance rather than to the law as a whole. For although women were largely barred from holding public office, even in the thirteenth century and earlier women were the equals of men in most aspects of private law. Records show them in various positions of power — as land-holders, for example; buying, selling, and renting their land; and conducting their own lawsuits. On closer inspection of the evidence,

'The distinction between public law and private law in mediaeval times shows unmistakably two worlds for women: the public world of modesty, silence, subjection and rightlessness; and the private world of responsibility for children and household, of rights to property and a hearing at law, of authority over children and of assertiveness in commercial dealings, no less than in marital discussion and decision.'   (Mount 1982:241)

Indeed, throughout the Middle Ages, evidence of endless and often wearisome debates about who should rule the household suggests the existence of an alternative pattern of marriage in which there was a high degree of equality between husband and wife. Furthermore, there were many variations on the prevailing orthodoxy of family life; many households were ruled by widows, whilst in others, at various times, men were away at war, and there was a persistent and sizeable number of 'common-law' marriages.

A rather different picture of the reality of marital and family experience has therefore emerged. The evidence, as far as it goes in shedding light on the historical ephemera of human relationships, tends to show that the *ideals* of love and equality were both present in the popular view of marriage; also that, amongst the population in general, to be happily married was always seen as one of the most important pieces of good fortune that life could offer. The fact that the commonly supposed transition from the traditional extended family towards the nuclear family now seems more doubtful, however, should not blind us to the fact that massive social, economic, and demographic changes occurred in Britain with the rise of capitalism and the ascendancy of Victorian morality, in its broadest sense, which had a profound effect upon the family and marriage. Nevertheless, Smelser (1982) has pointed out that there were many types of Victorian family, with one of the main factors underlying these variations being, as always, social class; the notion of a model Victorian family as an homogeneous social phenomenon, the passing of which is mourned by some and rejoiced by others, also seems something of a myth.

The middle-class Victorian family, for example, was symbolized by 'coolness and distance even in the most intimate relations' (Smelser 1982:65), by suppression of sexuality, and by a sharp and clear split in sex roles, the place of the woman being seen clearly as in the home. In contrast, all members of the working-class family worked hard in order for the family to subsist. Women shared similar occupations and experiences to men – although perhaps with greater variations allowing the inclusion of household duties, moving in and out of, and around in, the labour force as the ages, needs, and earning capacities of their children changed. As a result, there was also an increased separation of the work and leisure activities of spouses, and this seems to have been the major change. The household or the family continued to be the crucial economic unit, although for married working-class women the separation of home and work and the emergence of a fundamental split in sex roles meant that their influence was increasingly confined to the domestic sphere (Scott and Tilly 1975). This was reflected in both the predominance of young single girls in the female labour force and the relative absence of older married women. By 1911, 69 per cent of all single women worked, but only 9.6 per cent of married women did so. Furthermore, as Eversley and Bonnerjea (1982) have shown, late-nineteenth-century Britain still had families that were productive units, as well as families consisting of a single male wage-earner at the head of his nuclear family, a large number of one-parent households, and large family-type households incorporating servants and aged single relatives.

The processes of economic growth and improvements in the distribution of wealth, the beginnings of state welfare, and a whole series of social, economic, political, and legal changes had an increasing impact on working-class family life, not least by substantially reducing its dependency on multiple wage-earners, especially children. This, in turn, contributed to a major transformation that has continued into the twentieth century with the gradual replacement of familial values with increasingly individualistic ones. It became possible for both society and individuals to increase the investment in children's education, which, amongst other things, has led to increased inter-generational social mobility and the new individualistic attitude commonly ascribed to the modern twentieth-century marriage and nuclear family.

Before pursuing the analysis completely into the twentieth century, it is useful to go back once more to look in a little more detail at another factor that lies at the very core of marital and family life: romantic love and sex. These are also surrounded by a powerful mythology, both in the sense of the widespread current concern about the alleged excesses of our so-called permissive society, and in the widely held belief that this is a recent phenomenon unknown to previous generations. As Gathorne-Hardy has succinctly observed, 'Every age imagines it is unique, and usually that it is uniquely lewd' (1981:26). The evidence for the existence of both romantic and passionate sexual love within marriage as early as the thirteenth century has already been referred to. But evidence suggests that there were subsequent sexual 'revolutions', such as those that supposedly occurred at the end of the sixteenth century during the Restoration, and in the eighteenth century, during which there was a substantial liberalization of sexual attitudes and behaviour, before the sexually repressed Victorian era. Even pornography, commonly thought of as an indication of our own 'uniquely lewd' and even degenerate society, was popular and available during these periods, appearing in the court of Charles II during the first 'revolution', and then again in the eighteenth century. John Cleland's novel *Fanny Hill*, which has only comparatively recently been re-popularized as an example of the idiom, first appeared in 1748.

> 'By the end of the eighteenth century a market existed for regular pornographic magazines to be successful . . . In 1756 John Shebbeare remarked how "every print shop has its windows stacked full with indecent prints to inflame desire through the eye".'
>
> (Gathorne-Hardy 1981:45–6)

These earlier sexual revolutions were, it seems, not restricted solely to the élite of society but extended also to substantial sections of the upper and middle classes.

It is probable that the public and published debate and evidence of these sexual revolutions have a tendency to distort the extent of the change. 'All the time, largely unaffected, the mass of the people, the calm 70%, go on behaving much as they have always done' (Gathorne-Hardy 1981:33). Attitudes and behaviour in areas of our lives as fundamental as sex, marriage, and the family do not change throughout society at a rate fast enough to justify the term 'revolution'. Nevertheless real and substantial changes in sexual behaviour and attitudes have taken place, particularly in post-war Britain, not so much because the behaviour and attitudes are new, but because for the first time in history the changes have not been restricted to the élite but have spread to all levels of society. Part of the explanation for this lies in the revolution in contraceptive technology. Contraception is by no means a new development; *coitus interruptus*, which is still widely used, has been practised for centuries, and the sheath had been available in some form, first made of linen and subsequently of sheep's gut, since 1564. But not until the late nineteenth century, after advances in rubber technology had led to the invention of the rubber sheath and subsequently the Dutch cap, did the middle classes widely accept family planning, since when the practice has spread slowly and unevenly through all classes, the evidence for which lies in the fact that the average family size falls steadily after 1881. This technological revolution has, of course, continued leading ultimately to the introduction of the contraceptive pill. In terms of change, the significance of these developments lies as much in the increased sexual freedom to which they led, allowing an almost complete separation of sexual pleasure and procreation, as in the potential for effective family planning.

By the end of the nineteenth century, therefore, a number of changes were under way affecting family size, household structure, roles within families, employment, and attitudes within marriages and families towards sex and children. This process has continued into the twentieth century and has shaped modern marriage and the nuclear family, towards which we must now turn our attention, whilst remembering whence it came and the extensive mythology that surrounds its history.

Modern marriage and the family

At the centre of the modern nuclear family is what is frequently referred to as the companionate marriage, a model of the marital relationship that has grown over the last two centuries, albeit slowly at first, but with gathering speed this century. Today romantic love is widely regarded as the only legitimate basis for marriage, which is the primary relationship for both sexual and emotional fulfilment and personal growth, a subject that will be returned to later. The amazing success of modern medicine and community health-care policies in virtually eliminating death amongst children and young adults has also helped to transform the whole character of marriage and family life. The roles of parents in relation to their children have been profoundly altered. The rise of the meritocracy in employment has reduced family influence on job placement; the influence of parents on the marriage choices of their children has, with the exception of marriages amongst some ethnic minority groups, all but disappeared; in general there has been an erosion of patriarchal authority of husband over wife and of fathers over children; influenced by the work of writers such as Spock, Winnicott, and Bowlby, the family has become more child-centred, and child-rearing has become comparatively more permissive; children mature earlier sexually, but remain in full-time education and live at home longer than every before.

Stone (1977) has characterized the modern nuclear family as self-centred, inwardly turned, emotionally bonded, sexually liberated, and child-orientated. In addition to these many changes in family life, other broader social and demographic trends have had a massive impact on marriage and the family.

THE INSTITUTION OF MARRIAGE

During the twentieth century there has been a steady increase in the popularity of marriage and a steady decrease in age at first marriage, with marriage becoming so popular that it is attempted by almost everyone. This trend has slackened in the last decade. Since the early 1970s annual first marriage rates have fallen steadily, especially for those aged under twenty-five. In addition, the average age at marriage which reached an all-time low in 1970, has since started to rise (Leete 1976). The exact reasons for this are unclear and may include increased cohabitations, changing attitudes towards marriage in younger generations, and economic changes making early marriage more difficult. A growing surplus of males in the marriage market will in future result in the proportion of males remaining unmarried greatly exceeding that of females, although the higher the social class for men, the higher the proportion ultimately marrying (Haskey 1983c). In spite of these changes, Leete concludes that the majority of the population will marry at some time in their lives and that 'if as appears probable, there is a tendency to later marriage for recent generations, then the proportions of those generations who will eventually marry may not change very much at all' (1979:25)

The effect of cohabitation upon marriage has already been alluded to. Such relationships have always existed alongside formal marriages, and, as Brown and Kiernan have pointed out, 'there is good evidence that in Britain stable, long-lasting non-marital procreative unions in earlier periods (going back for several centuries) often attained the status of legal marriage' (1981:7). The Finer Committee on One-Parent Families argued that 'At no time in our history has it been so easy to obtain the sexual and other comforts of marriage without troubling to enter the institution' (DHSS 1974: vol.1, para.2.4, 6). There certainly is evidence of an increase in cohabitation. Dunnell (1979) reported that only 1 per cent of women first married between 1955 and 1960 cohabited with their husbands-to-be, but of those married between 1971 and 1975 this had increased to 9 per cent, with 14 per cent of women aged over twenty-five doing so, whilst some 3 per cent of single, widowed, divorced, or separated women were living with someone, two-fifths of these regarding themselves as married.

A similar picture was revealed by Brown and Kiernan (1981), who found 3 per cent of their sample of women cohabiting, with over half referring to themselves as 'married'. Their conservative estimate is that about a third of a million women aged under fifty are cohabiting, and that divorced and separated cohabiting women are much more likely to present themselves as married. Dunnell (1979), however, found that the length of pre-marital cohabitations was fairly short, with over a quarter of such relationships lasting less than three months, and nearly two-thirds lasting less than a year. In all, only 15 per cent of such relationships lasted for two years or longer, and the figures indicate that in a significant proportion of such relationships one or other party is not free to marry, although this is the expected eventual outcome. Whilst cohabitation has increased, therefore, the evidence does not suggest that it is seen as an alternative to marriage, but as an intervening stage between being single, or separated and awaiting divorce, and eventual marriage.

There have been important changes in family formation as a result of the immense progress in contraceptive technology. Whilst Dunnell (1979) found an increase in pre-marital sexual intercourse with future husbands, an increasing length of such sexual relationships, and an increase in the amount of cohabitation, Leete (1979) found that births conceived outside marriage are falling and that marriage remains the dominant institution within which child-bearing occurs. Nor, according to Dunnell, is there any clear sign that increasing proportions of women expect to remain childless or to have only one child, although there has been a definite trend this century towards smaller families; these are now the norm, although this varies with factors such as social class and ethnicity.

Along with the post-1970 trend towards later marriages, there has been a trend to delay the birth of the first child and to compress child-bearing into the first ten years of marriage, so women are able to return to work at an earlier age. Dunnell found that couples in the lower socio-economic classes marry younger and start their families earlier than couples higher up in the social scale. Although a higher proportion of women in the lower socio-economic classes were pregnant at marriage, after five years of marriage 70 per cent of all women had had one or two children, and the main class differences in this respect had disappeared. Dunnell suggests that there is a link between delaying marriage and/or the first child and expecting or desiring home ownership, which is a more common expectation in the higher socio-economic classes and raises the importance of economic factors in relation to marriage and the family (Dunnell 1979).

EMPLOYMENT

Dunnell (1979) found that, at the time of marriage, both home ownership and the extent to which expectations in relation to furniture and things for a home had been realized were directly related to socio-economic class. Income, both real and potential, is clearly important.

The fact that women in non-manual occupations waited longer after their marriage before their first child than those in manual jobs, and that those in professional and managerial jobs were much more likely to remain childless, points to the way in which the issue of employment enters into the most profound and intimate aspects of married life. Thus the entire increase in the working population between 1961 and 1975 is accounted for by the increase in the number of women by 30 per cent, from 7.7 million to 9.8 million (Central Statistical Office 1979, Table 5.1). During the recent recession, the number in employment fell from over 21.5 million in 1972, to just over 20.5 million in 1982, but the proportion of women increased from 38 to 43 per cent (Central Statistical Office 1984). By the early 1970s over 40 per cent of all married women worked. The majority were over thirty years old with children aged over eleven and were employed only part-time (Brayshaw 1980).

The picture that emerges is that the dual-career families studied by Rapoport and Rapoport (1976) are not typical of families in which wives work. There are variations in the general picture – for example, a higher proportion of professionally qualified mothers are employed compared with others, and amongst ethnic minority groups West Indian mothers are more likely to work outside the home than others. But the typical working wife is a middle-aged woman working part-time, generally at a job with very limited career prospects. In spite of the importance of the increase in economic power and freedom of women, indicating a growing equality between the sexes, the general predominance of the husband's employment and his usually greater earning power tend to ensure that it is the wife who reverts to the role of carer when necessary.

Another aspect of employment and the family is the reverse side of the coin: unemployment, redundancy, early retirement, and youth unemployment. All these have increased in recent years and have a major impact on family life, which will be referred to in the next chapter. All these facts, however, suggest that, in some ways at least, the family as an economic unit is experiencing something of a renaissance, across class boundaries, and that the justification for married women working today is not so different from that proposed for working married women in the eighteenth and nineteenth centuries. A study by Rossiter (1980) tends to confirm this view, showing that the main reason for women seeking work outside the home is money – over 70 per cent of her sample – rather than self-fulfilment or other similar reasons (see also Sharpe 1984).

DIVORCE

No attempt at analysing and understanding modern marriage and family life can avoid an examination of what is perhaps the single most significant social trend in post-war Britain: the steady escalation of the divorce rate. The increased ease of divorce as a result of progressive changes in the law and the increased availability of legal aid are frequently pointed to as important factors, since such changes are clearly associated with rises in the divorce rate. But as Leete (1979) has pointed out, these are short-term effects, and the underlying upward movement has continued. The scale of the trend is described by Chester as

> 'a contemporary mass phenomenon of considerable social import-ance, and some observers have deduced from them a substantial decline in the stability of marriage. Unless, however, marital stability is to be measured by the mere maintenance of the legal tie, such a conclusion goes somewhat beyond existing evidence.'   (1972:529)

Chester goes on to argue the need for caution in interpreting divorce statistics, in view of the potential for incremental inaccuracies, which can progressively distort the final figure for marriages that end in divorce. Such statistics remain a very crude indicator of the extent of marital disruption, let alone marital satisfaction and happiness. Dunnell (1979) suggests that in the 1960s the divorce statistics showed only about one-half of total marriage breakdowns. Although with more liberal divorce laws this discrepancy is now likely to be less than before, caution is still required in dealing with divorce data.

The presentation of figures also creates confusion, distortions, and even anxiety. Haskey, for example, predicts that 'approximately 1 in 3 marriages may be expected to end in divorce if divorce rates conti-nue at their current levels' (1982:5), creating an impression of an epi-demic of divorcing couples and broken families. The same facts, presented by Haskey in a different way, put the rate in 1980 at 12 divorces per 1,000 marriages; whilst it is hard to be complacent about the fact that this is twice the rate of 1971 and three times the rate of 1968, the impact on the reader is somewhat different. Similarly, Dun-nell records that in 1978 nearly 163,000 children under sixteen were involved in divorce, so that 'we might expect that between 1 in 5 and 1 in 6 children born today may witness their parents' divorce before they reach 16' (1979:36) – a figure confirmed by Haskey (1983a). Whilst the implications of such figures are enormous, this represents only 13 out of every 1,000 children in that age group in any year (Leete 1979:95).

Certain factors are nevertheless associated with the divorce rate, and there is common agreement that age at marriage – especially of the wife – and duration of marriage are key variables (Dunnell 1979, Haskey 1982 and 1983b, Leete 1979, Rimmer 1981). Divorce rates reach a peak for couples between the ages of 25 and 29, and divorce is occurring after progressively shorter periods of marriage. Rimmer (1981) shows that 30 per cent of all divorces, the largest single group, are from marriages of between 5 and 9 years' duration; and recent figures from Haskey (1982) show that the highest rate of divorce now occurs after only three years of marriage. Young marriages in general, and teenage marriages in particular, are more divorce prone, whilst teenage brides who are pregnant at marriage are more likely to experience marital breakdown than any other group of women.

Differences between groups drawn on other lines, such as socio-economic class, are, surprisingly, harder to determine; as Chester comments, 'The official statistics do not routinely report on this variable' (1972:537). It seems likely, however, that more than 80 per cent of divorces now occur in marriages in which the husband is below social classes I and II, and that within this, class V – i.e. unskilled workers – is over-represented. 'At some uncertain, but relatively recent point, then, the working class seems to have surpassed the higher status groups in contribution to divorce' (Chester 1972:537). Probably, at least in part, this is a result of the greater legal and economic availability of divorce. There is little doubt therefore that marital instability, at least as reflected by divorce rates, is inversely related to social class.

Evidence relating to ethnicity and divorce is even more scarce. Although

> 'there is some evidence to suggest that slightly more West Indian families have only one parent – 13% in 1976 compared with 9% of all families – whereas only 1% of Asian families were headed by a lone parent at that date'   (Rimmer 1981:38)

such figures must be treated with great caution. At least part of the explanation may lie, for example, in different patterns of family formation amongst West Indian communities (Driver 1982, Foner 1977).

Whilst such an upward surge in divorce rates is a comparatively recent phenomenon, it is almost universal in the West and it seems unlikely to be temporary or transient. Chester argues that high levels of marital instability

'should be expected to become a normal feature of social experience . . . it is difficult to find any theoretical reason or empirical
evidence to suggest that the recent upward trend is due for
reversal.'   (1972:533)

REMARRIAGE

It would be erroneous to assume that the rising divorce rate indicates
disillusionment with marriage as an institution, or that divorce is a
matter of fashion (Brayshaw 1980:11). This would be to trivialize
both marriage – and the idealism and striving with which it is almost
universally invested by those who undertake it – and divorce, with the
anguish and suffering frequently experienced by those who resort to
it. Indeed, as the figures above indicate and as Gathorne-Hardy
observes, 'the institution of marriage still rests on a bedrock of statistical stability' (1981:156). However,

> 'the idea of divorce is inherent in the ideal of companionate mar-
> riage. If the main aim of marriage is companionship and mutual
> help, then once that ceases there is no point in continuing it.'
> (Gathorne-Hardy 1981:151)

Given that the ideal of the companionate marriage is a powerful
social reality, and that the new ideology of personal growth and fulfilment through the ideal of romantic sexual love in marriage is a major
factor in this, it is not surprising to find, along with high rates of divorce,
high rates of remarriage. Leete (1979) has concluded that younger first
marriages, together with younger divorce, have led to younger age at
remarriage, so that currently around one-third of divorced people who
are under thirty remarry each year. This in turn suggests that a high
proportion of those who divorce before the age of thirty, though not
all, will remarry within a few years of divorce, and that substantially
more than one-third of those now divorcing will eventually remarry.
Rimmer (1981) has noted one factor that seems to influence the
proportion of remarrying women: the age of the youngest child at divorce. Those whose youngest child was under ten remarry more often
than those whose children are older, or indeed than those who had no
children. She suggests that one interpretation of this is that it may
reflect the attitudes of children towards step-parents, with older
children being more reluctant to accept them, which in turn might
affect the mother's attitude towards remarriage. Such mothers are

also more likely to be younger than those with older children and therefore more likely to remarry in any event. A further element of explanation may lie in the severe economic hardship faced by many one-parent families after divorce and therefore the existence of purely economic pressures towards remarriage, since children in step-families 'were far less likely to live in or below the poverty line than those in one-parent families' (Eekelaar and Maclean 1983:31). Thus, whilst the affective rewards of modern family life are seen by many as being of at least equal and possibly even greater importance than the instrumental rewards, and are at the heart of the ideals held by many of their own marriages, the nuclear family and the companionate marriage within it still retain a firm identity as an economic as well as social unit.

The step-family therefore is an increasingly common form of the family today. In view of the disruption, for both adults and children, surrounding marital breakdown and divorce, however, it is perhaps sad, in terms of the human cost, to find that remarriages are not necessarily the solution to the problems that led to the first divorces of the remarried couple. Rimmer notes that

'the proportion of divorces involving re-divorce for one or both partners has risen from under 9% in 1966 to 16% in 1979 . . . .Today, then, 1 in 20 divorces involves re-divorce for both partners.' (1981:47)

This trend is confirmed by Haskey (1983b). What is more, Leete (1979) observes that divorcing for a second time and marrying for a third time are also becoming less uncommon. The step-family as a result of divorce is thus as prevalent today as the step-family as a result of death was in previous eras.

THE FAMILY LIFE CYCLE

The mistake of historians in failing to take into account variations in family structure resulting from different stages in the family life cycle has already been referred to, and this applies equally to the modern family. It is widely recognized that another major demographic change, with far-reaching effects at all levels of society, is taking place as a result of our ageing population. Even as recently as 1901 the life expectancy of a boy and girl born in that year would have been only 48 and 52 years respectively, whereas now it is 70 and 76 respectively. Rimmer (1981) found that three-quarters of women over the age of eighty-five who were living without their husbands but with 'others' are living with either their children or their children-in-law, as are four-fifths of men living without their wives. She also found that the most frequent visitors to elderly people are their children or children-in-law, and that it is to their families that many people turn for help in their old age (Rimmer 1981: 57–8; see also Nissel 1982).

The significance of this should not be missed, in terms of either its impact on marital and family life or the alleged selfish, uncaring, and insular nature of the modern nuclear family. As Eversley and Bonnerjea (1982) point out, it has been argued that, ever since the advent of the first Poor Law in 1601, the family has progressively lost or been deprived of its caring functions, most especially in the post-Beveridge era of social policy and reform. Evidence such as Rimmer's (1981) however, tends to emphasize the increasing importance of the caring role of the family in relation to the elderly, whilst there is similar evidence of its caring role in relation to physical and mental health, educational attainment, and many other areas of family life. Similarly, as Mount says, 'All the evidence . . . suggests that people see *more* of their non-resident kin – parents, aunts, and uncles – not less than they used to' (1982:168) – a view confirmed by Rapoport and Rapoport (1982).

At the other end of the family cycle, the practice of sharing homes with in-laws after marriage is still widespread. Immediately after marriage, just over a quarter of all couples share homes, almost all with parents, whilst a similar proportion rent from private landlords (Brayshaw 1980). In order to achieve the almost universally sought-after goal of marriage, then, more than half of newly married couples are prepared to put up with unsatisfactory housing arrangements. So at both ends of the family life cycle, the extended multi-generational family still exists in Britain today, probably to much the same extent as it ever did. As Nissel has said, 'Social change has different effects on families and individuals within families at different stages of the life cycle' (1982:95).

Summary

What has been offered in the preceding pages, as a prelude to an examination of the problems faced by marriages today, has been a brief exploration of the history of marriage in Britain and of its family context, in order to shed some light on the mythology surrounding it. As Pincus and Dare have observed,

'The concept of myth is not easy to define: we can use it to describe a falsification of a situation or we can use it to mean stories or legends which reveal rather than hide essential underlying truths.'   (1978:9)

In this case, the essential underlying truth that is revealed is the nature of our ideals and aspirations for marriage and family. Since these are derived substantially from our perceptions of history, this must be properly understood if modern marriage is to be fully comprehended.

Similarly:

'A myth, of course, is not a fairy story. It is the presentation of facts belonging to one category in the idioms appropriate to another. To explore a myth is accordingly not to deny the facts but to re-allocate them.'

(Ryle, 'The Concept of Mind', quoted in Pearson 1983:205)

Just such a re-allocation of facts has been sought. It has become apparent that various historical distortions have intruded into and obscured our commonly held views, beliefs, and understanding about marriage and the family in times past. As Scott and Tilly have argued, 'We must examine *their* experience in the light of their familial values and not our own individualistic ones' (1975:178).

Thus the supposed earlier 'golden age', when marriages and families were stable and enduring, emerges substantially as a myth. Although this myth may reflect important ideals, it may also lead to unrealistically high expectations of and demands on marriage today. At the level of family structure, we also find discrepancies between belief and fact, leading Laslett, amongst others, to the inescapable conclusion that 'The wish to believe in the large and extended house-hold as the ordinary institution of an earlier England . . . is indeed a matter of ideology' (1972a:73). And Mount has reasoned:

'If the evidence we have put together is correctly interpreted, the family as we know it today – small, two generation, nuclear, based on choice and affection . . . – is neither a novelty, nor the product of unique historical forces.'   (1982:153)

Pursuing this same theme of mythology and ideology, Pearson suggests that in the light of such historical distortions

'The recurring allegations against the decline of the family must also invite suspicion . . . . The historical record registers centuries of complaint against weakened family ties . . . [but] the family today is stronger – both as a material force and as an ideology – than at any time in remembered history.'   (1983:210–11)

What of marriage and the family as we know them today? It is perhaps ironic that, in his attempts to dismantle the mythology of the family in history, Mount (1982) appears to accept the myth of the modern nuclear family; for, as the facts about the modern family suggest, the commonly held model of the typical nuclear family unit, consisting of a couple and their children living together in their own home, is in some senses as unrealistic as the model of the traditional extended family. Such families make up about a third of households at any one time. If the model is even more rigid – with father as the bread-winner at the head of the family, and mother at home – this would apply to only about 15 per cent of households; and if only natural parents were included the proportion would be smaller still. Therefore as Rimmer comments, 'Even though the majority of parents, children and families still follow a fairly traditional pattern the minority who do not is growing' (1981:63).

Whilst the conventional family may increasingly be a myth statistically speaking at any given time, however, it is a reality for many at some point in the family life cycle (Chester 1985a). It is widely regarded as a norm and an ideal to be striven for, with many people apparently viewing marriage and parenthood not only as inseparable, but also as inevitable and desirable. This is why the family has been considered in some detail alongside marriage in this and subsequent chapters.

The comparison has revealed a remarkable number of similarities between traditional and modern marriages and families, some of which will be pursued further in the next chapter. Patterns of husbands' and wives' employment have long had, and continue to have, a profound impact on marital relationships and the division of marital roles; poverty and housing continue to exert a powerful influence on marital relationships and choices; whilst children and families are a major consideration and influence in the lives of most couples. Romantic love and affection have always been associated in varying degrees with marriage and couple relationships. Divorce and marital breakdown are not a phenomenon associated solely with marriage in the post-war years. Family life has always been disrupted – in the past by death, now by divorce – and the step-family and one-parent family are not new arrivals on the social scene. Moreover, the notion that the instability of modern marriages and families makes society itself more unstable seems hard to sustain, since social stability depends on the fact that socialization and cultural transmission can continue, despite death or divorce, and the high rate of remarriage makes this possible.

But neither must we be blind to the differences between traditional and modern patterns. Today, for example, when families split the children are usually young, whilst in pre-industrial Britain, when death was the major cause of remarriage, the reverse was true. The notion of divorce as a functional substitute for death, whilst interesting, tends not to be supported by the evidence of higher rates of divorce in the early years of marriage. There has been what Mount describes as 'a simple, once-for-all jump from divorce controlled by the State and the Church to divorce controlled by the married couple' (1982:216). There have been widespread changes in sexual behaviour and attitudes. These are not, it has been suggested, as recent as is commonly supposed, and it can be argued that the changes often attributed to the social and sexual revolution of the post-war years are often essentially ones of expression. None the less, such changes as have occurred are spread more widely throughout society than ever before. Perhaps, more subtly, it must be recognized that, especially in post-war Britain,

'Romantic love, providing a respectable, age-old, glorifying ideology for natural sexual restlessness, attained immeasurable physical gravitational force by drawing into itself things as fundamental as children, marriage and "growth".' (Gathorne-Hardy 1981:146)

Paradoxically, this can be regarded as by far the most important cause of marital breakdown. For it can be argued that romantic love and marriage are incompatible – with marriage being based upon closeness, familiarity, and mutual ease, whilst romantic love is a distant quest, the exploration of something new, feeding upon feelings that are enhanced by partings and obstacles. Thus, it is suggested, the natural and even desirable attrition of romantic love by the reality of the developing marital relationship may induce conflicting feelings: anxiety; fear of failure; desperation at the disappearance of the feelings associated with the romantic love that first drew and held two people together; and despair at the prospect of regularity, familiarity, and mutuality, extending into an undifferentiated future of married boredom. New, extramarital relationships offer adventure, the rediscovery of romantic love, or, perhaps for some, more prosaically, simple relief from boredom. Whatever the merits of this argument, however, the significance of the ideology and mythology of romantic love for marriage today must not be lost.

Whilst there are many continuities, therefore, there have also been important changes in marriage and the family and in the broader social background against which modern marriages and families are made. The separate trends of many of these changes have been evident for some time. Gathorne-Hardy suggests:

'The causes of the present situation . . . lie in a vast complex of social, historical, physical, legal, psychological and technological forces – some recent, some very ancient – which have all come together in a peculiarly intense way over the last thirty years.'   (1981:300)

The attitudes, values, and beliefs that we all hold about marriage and the family are crucial in shaping our perception of the situations we encounter. Some understanding of their historical origin and validity is essential if social-work intervention with marital problems is to be effective. Although we are concerned with marital problems, these are often closely interwoven with the fabric of family life and of society. Indeed, many marital problems come to the attention of social workers only as a result of family problems, and social work has been involved with families and their problems since it first emerged out of the rapid social and economic changes of the last century. The next task is to explore the problems that some of the most significant of these changes have created for marriage and the family.

2
Problems in marital relationships

As we have argued in the previous chapter, marriage and family life are undergoing perhaps the most far-reaching processes of change they have ever known. This is in part the result of a wide and complex array of social changes, but also because of a reappraisal of the meaning of marriage and consequent changes in expectations of it. To these social, economic, and interpersonal factors, and their contribution to the creation of problems in marriage, must be added the intrapersonal factors that have always been important in influencing the marital relationship. The aim of this chapter is to explore the nature of the evidence about marital problems, since an awareness of such evidence must be an important factor in the ability of social workers to be sensitive to and aware of the existence of marital problems in the lives of their clients, and the ways such problems might be generated.

There are two major difficulties in attempting to achieve such an understanding. First, whilst we know a great deal about marriage from a vast array of social research that has looked at marriage from the outside, we do not in fact know much – other than from our own personal experience – about the reality of marriages from the inside. Mount has commented: 'It is the essence of marriage that it is private and apart from the rest of society. Its "selfishness" or "exclusiveness" is not its undertone but its heart and soul' (1982:188). We are faced with a similar problem to that with which we grappled in Chapter 1: how to put the emotional flesh on the bare bones of fact, and how to allocate the facts correctly. The second major problem is how to understand the facts about divorce and marital breakdown and their relationship with happiness and satisfaction in marriage. The latter must be of concern to social workers if they are to be able to identify problems and to consider intervention, whether this be in terms of sustaining the relationship or of facilitating disengagement from it. As Chester has reasoned, there may even be arguments for people to change spouses when appropriate in order to maximize personal satisfactions:

> 'Certainly it is not clear that all therapeutic intervention should concentrate on the prevention of breakup to the exclusion of action to minimise any individually disruptive consequences there may be when breakup does occur.'   (1972:540)

We refer to this subject later in the book (see Chapter 8).

In seeking to understand the facts we possess, we must accept that divorce is not an accurate indicator of dissatisfaction in marriage. Conflicts and tension are not necessarily indicative of marital instability, even though couples may experience them as problematic. Indeed, it is likely that only a few marriages of any length will have completely avoided conflict or relationship difficulties, although the extent to which these are seen as 'marital problems' is a different matter. Gathorne-Hardy has observed:

> 'The most neurotic, the most difficult marriages, those with a lot of anger and frustration, are not those that dissolve most easily. In fact, outwardly bad marriages often last till death. It is the easy marriages . . . that often separate so smoothly they scarcely seem to have been joined.'   (1981:295)

Empirical support for this contention is provided by Hicks and Platt: 'Perhaps the single most provocative finding is that low happiness may often be associated with marital stability' (1970:569); the strength of the marital bond can be only partially assessed by the variable of 'marital happiness'. Chester (1980), in a wide-ranging review of the literature on marital problems, concludes that a high proportion of modern marriages do experience problems of one kind or another, but that accurate measurement is difficult since the bulk of research has concentrated on statistics relating to marital breakdown. Since these facts have already been outlined, we must now examine some of the scattered and predominantly American studies that might increase our understanding of marital problems.

Marital satisfaction and the family life cycle

The concept of the family life cycle has attracted a considerable amount of research attention. The importance of this in relation to understanding the reality of marital and family relationships has already been argued in Chapter 1, whilst Nissel (1982) has demonstrated in some detail how the changes of recent decades have had varying impacts upon families at different stages in their life cycle. The consensus of United States research (e.g. Figley 1973, Glenn and Weaver 1978, Rollins and Cannon 1974, Ryder 1973), following the development of a model of the family life cycle by Duvall (1967), is that marital satisfaction tends to decline from initial high levels during the early years of marriage, to a low point in the final stages of the child-bearing phase of family life, when there are teenaged children at home. After this it increases again, although this may be mediated by an intervening factor such as role strain, which appears to be related to both marital satisfaction and family life cycle. The only analogous British research, reported by Walker, revealed a broadly similar picture, but suggested that the British wife is

> 'least satisfied with the expressive components of married life . . . . She expects more in the way of companionship, in the amount of understanding of the way she feels and in the expressions of love than she presently receives, though she is relatively more satisfied with material aspects of the marriage and with her experience of motherhood.'   (Walker 1977:134)

Implicit in this view, once again, is the ideal of personal fulfilment through the experience of romantic love in the context of a companionate marriage.

Whilst the concept of the family life cycle as a research tool is problematic, Chester concludes that 'Although currently much may not be known about it, there clearly is some kind of time dimension in the course of marital problems and marital instability' (1980:89). The value of this approach lies in providing a framework within which certain events, roles, tasks, and problems will predictably occur for many married couples. Authors such as Carter and McGoldrick (1980) have adopted this framework for the more systematic practice of family therapy. With the aim of providing more of a descriptive framework, Dominian (1980) has proposed a simpler model, which will be used as a basis for exploring problems in the marital relationship.

32 Couples, conflict, and change

Dominian sees this phase as spanning approximately the first five years of marriage, until the couple are in their late twenties or early thirties, although the background to and the start of the relationship seem as important to consider as the event of marriage. In the case of remarriages and step-families, different parameters may need to be adopted, since such marriages will occur at different ages and will experience only part-cycles or irregular cycles. A weak relationship has been noted (Bumpass and Sweet 1972, Mueller and Pope 1977) between parental divorce and divorce in the children of such marriages, which from the outset become more liable to disruption and divorce than others; but Thornes and Collard concluded on the basis of their findings that 'There appeared to be no general link between parental bond breaking *per se* and offspring marital bond breaking' (1979:17). This point was echoed by Chester (1980:104) after a review of the evidence.

Thornes and Collard (1979) did find, however, that some background factors were positively associated with eventual divorce: e.g. those marriages in which the wife had been an only child, those in which the husband had grown up without a sister, those preceded by short courtships, or without any informal engagement or honeymoon, those towards which there was strong opposition (usually parental), and those in which there were more break-ups in the relationship preceding marriage. Ineichen (1977) found that shorter courtship periods were also associated with teenage brides. Factors preceding marriage are thus of considerable importance. Thornes and Collard also found that, although this early period of marriage seems to be critically related to marital stability, 'When their serious marital problems started, the couples did not quickly separate, and marital difficulties, which frequently started very early in the marriage, tended to be tolerated for quite long periods' (1979:129) – which at the very least allows time for attempts to be made to resolve them.

Amongst the social tasks faced by the married couple in this first phase Dominian (1980) includes the process of detachment from parents and friends and the development of an inward focus. This may include some combination of previously separate leisure activities, all of which will be, to some extent, a continuation of the adjustments begun during courtship in terms of learning new roles (a subject that will be returned to later – see pp. 39–41), creating new networks, or revising old ones. The social tasks also include establishing a viable interpersonal relationship, setting up a home, supporting it financially whilst sharing the tasks involved in running it, and, for many, combining two working lives. Evidently, at this level alone, the tasks are many and complex, and the potentiality for problems is great. Ineichen (1977) has argued that in young marriages the combination of youth and other related problems – e.g. a relatively weak financial situation and inferior housing arrangements, with just over one-half of couples starting married life with relatives compared with just under a quarter of older wives, and with fewer becoming owner-occupiers and many more becoming council tenants – amounts to 'a vortex of disadvantage', a picture confirmed by Madge and Brown (1981). Much of the explanation for this is the strong connections between age, earnings, and occupational class. Whilst such problems are not necessarily typical, they throw into sharp relief the problems many newly married couples face to one degree or another.

Dominian (1980) also draws attention to the physical side of marriage during the early years and the importance of sexual adjustment. Thornes and Collard (1979), for example, found that 10 to 20 per cent of couples experienced some initial sexual dissatisfaction. A process of mutual sharing and learning needs to occur if this adjustment is to be successfully made, and ignorance, even of basic physiological facts, may well make an impact. Problems such as non-consummation, premature ejaculation, and partial or complete impotence on the part of the husband may occur. The wife may fail to enjoy sex or to experience orgasm, perhaps as a result of an inability to relax because of high levels of tension, or fear of pregnancy, whilst either may experience an inability to combine notions of romantic love with a physical relationship. Emotional tasks and an ability to adjust to both physical and emotional intimacy are also of central importance, requiring

> 'and increasing level of sensitive awareness, accurate response, empathy, the ability to express and register affection and the feeling that the couple matter to each other. Common difficulties at this stage of marriage are the failure of adequate communication and insufficient time spent together.'   (Dominian 1980:23)

These two problems in particular can occur at any stage of a marriage, but the tasks involved are particularly important during the early years because of what Dominian describes as 'The transition from falling in love to loving' (1980:23). Whilst the effects of assortive mating result in most spouses having similar educational and intellectual backgrounds, this alone cannot guarantee that such emotional communication will occur, nor that there will necessarily be shared standards and values in relation to finances, political outlook, child-rearing, and other important areas of married life, and most couples will need to work on the evolution of these.

As Dominian has observed,

> 'The arrival of the first child is one of the most important events in this phase of marriage. The couple now become a triad; the wife has to learn how to be a wife—mother; the husband, husband—father.'   (1980:24)

Significantly, many spouses with marital problems identify the birth of a child as the time at which these began. Research in the United States on the impact of children on the marital relationship (e.g. Figley 1973, Glenn and McLanahan 1982, Glenn and Weaver 1978, Hobbs and Cole 1976, Lerner and Spanier 1976, Miller 1976, Ryder 1973) leads to the overwhelming conclusion that the arrival of children brings with it a disruptive and potentially difficult transition; and for many, children have a negative impact on marital satisfaction. In Britain, Thornes and Collard (1979) reached similar conclusions. They found that divorcing couples seemed more likely than those continuing with their marriages to have had a child within two years of the wedding, particularly in the first year of marriage. Amongst the vast majority of divorced couples, the difficulties had arisen when the wife was still involved with infant care.

The nature of the difficulties caused by the arrival of children is multi-faceted. Children take time and energy that might otherwise be devoted to supporting the couple relationship, and their presence not only intrudes into this intimate interaction but creates a more complex social system, with greater potential for conflict and disagreement over issues related to child-rearing. It may also be that many new parents are ill-prepared for their new roles and responsibilities, to which husband and wife may react differently, leading to a divergence of previously shared perspectives on marriage. Husbands may begin to extend their activities outside the home, whilst wives may have to give up work, with all the social, economic, and psychological changes to which that may give rise. For both, there will be a disruption of social, domestic, and sexual life to varying degrees. Little wonder then that such a transition can result in a level of stress that ultimately leads to the break-up of many marriages, especially if we recall the emphasis in modern marriage on personal fulfilment through the ideal of romantic love.

Thus we have uncovered yet another myth in relation to marriage:

the predominant belief that children represent the ultimate fulfilment in marriage leading to happiness and stability, a belief that contributes to the fact that 90 per cent of married couples become parents, and that childlessness for most is involuntary. In addition to such positive social pressures towards parenthood, Chester (1980) argues the existence of a cultural negative stereotype of childless couples; this can generate problems of various kinds for a marriage, resulting from feelings of stigmatization and almost of deviance, and from pressures from family and friends. Involuntary childlessness may induce feelings of failure in women who cannot conceive or in men who are infertile, which may lead to stress on all aspects of the marriage. Medical treatment, perhaps lasting for some time, may be involved. A sex life overshadowed by temperature charts and ovulation cycles inevitably loses some of its spontaneity, since it becomes an activity that can no longer be enjoyed for itself – as most couples have come to expect – but one that is simply engaged in for the purpose of procreation.

Francis (1984b) has argued that, with 1 in 7 couples now seeking help over problems in conceiving a child, and 1 couple in 15 permanently childless, a considerable need is emerging for infertility counselling and an awareness amongst social workers of the emotional difficulties arising from childlessness. Perhaps as a result of these factors, recent evidence shows that childless marriages are more divorce-prone, although Chester (1985b) points out that this is also associated with above-average fertility. Indeed, Houseknecht (1979) found some evidence in the United States that women who were childless by choice had a better overall level of marital adjustment than mothers; whilst, in Britain, Humphrey (1975) found that husbands and wives who were childless consistently obtained higher affection scores than those with children, perhaps because childlessness can lead to closer mutual affinity in thoughts and feelings.

So the critical importance of the early years of marriage is reflected by the high rate of divorce in short-duration marriages. There are many adjustments to be made and problems to be overcome during this period, which not only provides the foundations for the ensuing phases of married life, but also the planting ground for the seeds of problems that might subsequently lead to marital unhappiness and instability.

PHASE 2: THE MIDDLE YEARS

This phase broadly covers couples aged between 30 and 50 and spans many years and many changes, the chronology of which is far from rigid. It is the phase in which most child-rearing activity takes place, ending when the children leave home. The research relating to the decline in marital satisfaction during this period of child-rearing has already been referred to, and clearly there will be different demands and problems depending, at least in part, on the number and ages of children. It is also a period in which personal growth continues, as a result of which Dominian suggests that partners may 'exhibit marked changes in their personality' (1980:24). Chester also observes that middle-age marriages

> 'are potentially under greater strain than at any time since the initial impact of having to accommodate to intimate life together. Married relationships are often somewhat hollow, having experienced gradual decline in sexual relations, companionship, demonstrations of affection, and sharing of interests.'   (1980:98-9)

Many of the problems that may be encountered by couples in this stage of their marriages are developments or continuations of those in the early years of married life. Some are specific to the middle years, however, such as various employment-related factors: e.g. the pressures of social mobility, either upward or downward, or even non-mobility. Many working husbands will have reached the limits of their career or employment potential and will have to adjust both to this and to diminishing physical resources, whilst many wives will return to work during this period.

As parents, the spouses will be facing the manifold problems of dealing with growing adolescent children who are struggling to find their own identity, not infrequently through challenging their parents, resulting in inter-generational conflict. Simultaneously, whilst sexual maturity is occurring at ever younger ages (having fallen by three years in the last hundred years), paradoxically the period of full entry into the adult world is being extended by the increasing duration of education, and other socio-economic factors such as unemployment and shortages of appropriate housing. The peer group has become almost as important as the family in the social life of teenaged children, and the emergence in post-war Britain of a more or less permanent, although changing, subculture of youth would seem to provide evidence of such changes. In addition, this period sees the eventual leaving home and often the marriage of children, with the readjustments necessitated by this – plus, for many, the advent of new problems if the spouses' own parents become frail or ill. The death of a parent, apart from the grief this may cause, may also create a problem of caring for the remaining parent if they too are frail or ill.

The physical side of marriage continues to be important during the middle years. Whilst Thornes and Collard (1979) found that the vast majority of continuing married men and women were satisfied with the sexual side of marriage, sexual problems do occur in this period:

> 'The statistics of marital breakdown ... show clearly that this is most likely early in marriage and considerably later, around 17 years after marriage. It is obvious that problems ... [of] the second group [are] likely to be related to children growing up, leaving home, the marriage partners being thrown back again on their own company and resources which may be severely strained.'
>
> (Crown 1976:259)

Additionally, sexual difficulties during this period may be a continuation of initial difficulties, or the result of problems emerging after childbirth, as well as those resulting from a general deterioration of the relationship.

Dominian believes that the emotional side of marriage assumes increasing importance in this phase of married life:

> 'In the intimacy of the contemporary marriage couples tend to experience one another as they have experienced the crucial encounters with their own parents, and in fact it can be said that there are two intimate experiences in life, the first between ourselves and our parents and the second with our spouses. In the first relationship trust, autonomy, initiative, self-esteem, the cycle of conflict-anger-guilt, envy and jealousy were all established and these patterns have a tendency to repeat themselves in the second and subsequent relationship.'
>
> (Dominian 1980:26)

This important perspective is of relevance at other stages in the marital relationship, but especially so in the middle years after the romantic intensity and passions of the early years of the relationship have been mellowed by the passage of time. A growth of independence out of earlier dependence may occur in the middle years, and the spouse who sought to transfer their dependency from their parents to their partner may grow in self-reliance and emerge as a person in their own right. Whilst many couples adjust to these changes, 'This asymmetrical growth from dependence to independence is a major psychological contribution to marital breakdown' (Dominian 1980: 27), especially if it coincides with some of the other problems outlined above.

PHASE 3: THE CONCLUDING YEARS

This phase covers marriage from the age of about fifty to its conclusion with the death of a spouse. Divorce is relatively uncommon at this stage of marriage, since divorce rates decline with the duration of marriage (Leete 1979). It may be tempting to infer that problems are unlikely because most marriages of this duration appear stable. As has already been argued, however, marital stability and happiness are not necessarily related, and important changes still occur.

For most marriages, children will have left home, leaving the original one-to-one marital relationship. With today's increased life expectancy, this phase of marriage may well last twenty years or longer, with the result that the management of age becomes an increasingly important issue. Initially, whilst couples are in their fifties, they often experience a renewed freedom to pursue either shared or solitary activities because health is not generally impaired; but from the sixties onwards there is an increased incidence of ill-health. Additionally, the dyadic marital relationship may once again be interrupted, only this time by the advent of an ageing parent (see, for example, Bowling 1984). In Britain, 80 per cent of the elderly live either in the same household as their children or less than half an hour's journey from them (Dominian 1980:28, Study Commission on the Family 1980:32). This phase also represents the period of retirement or redundancy, with all that this implies for many about reduced economic circumstances, and the need to adjust to a different socio-economic status and pattern of life.

There are also important aspects to the physical side of marriage during this phase. Its beginning sees the average age of the menopause in women, which Dominian suggests is often used as an excuse for sexual difficulties, although there is no evidence that it is, by itself, responsible for these. Often the menopause provides a convenient rationalization for existing difficulties. In addition, as Pitt suggests,

'Many people find the idea of sexual activity in later life distasteful . . . . Old people themselves, brought up at a time when sex was not a subject to be spoken of, are very slow to talk of their needs, especially to professional workers like doctors and social workers.'   (1976:297)

Whilst there is a general decline in sexual activity throughout adult life, with a sharp reduction in those over seventy-five, the decline in sexual interest, at least in men, is much less marked. The presence of a sexual partner, in conjunction with an active early sex life and good physical health, are all conducive to sexual activity in old age, although there are of course immense individual variations. Besides the general decline, age-specific impotency in men appears more frequently, with increasing age bringing increasing difficulties in developing an erection, penetration, and ejaculation. Also depression, a common disorder in the elderly, may well lead to reduced sexual drive and activity.

For many couples, this phase of married life is a rich and rewarding period, producing great comfort and security as a result of the close knowledge and communication that have been built up over the years. For others, however, with the departure of the children comes the realization that their marriage is little more than an empty shell in which they have lived their marriage through the children rather than through each other. Some of these marriages may break down, whilst others will linger on in a state of emotional neutrality or resigned unhappiness rather than face the uncertainties of old age alone.

Marriage ends, in physical terms, with the death of one of the spouses, usually the husband. However, grief-work and mourning apart, a marriage will often continue to have enormous psychological importance to an elderly person, since for many it represents their life's ambitions and their life's achievements. It is important to remember this coda therefore; to suggest that marriage does not end until the death of *both* spouses is to do more than just to romanticize the marital relationship in old age.

Structural issues

Our discussion of the life cycle of marriage and the family has highlighted some of the problems likely to occur at different stages. To a considerable extent, such problems are chronological and are intrinsic to the dynamic nature of marriage and family life. There are, however, a range of other issues that are related more to structural factors, both within and without marriage. These are of crucial importance not only in understanding and analysing marital relationships, but also in identifying other potential sources of difficulty.

One such area is the relationship between role perceptions, expectations, and marital happiness. Elizabeth Bott's (1971) seminal work, on the relationship between the degree of segregation of marital roles and the interconnectedness of couples' social networks, resulted in a substantial amount of interest in this particular aspect of the way marital relationships are structured. This particular approach will not be explored in detail here, although the significance of the insights offered should be noted. As Brannen and Collard suggest, the sets of intimate relationships which surround marriages 'are likely to determine, to some extent at least, how couples perceived and acted out their marital relationships and the problems that these came up against' (1982:111). Similarly, Rapoport and Rapoport, discussing the supposed erosion of family support networks, have commented: 'What has been stressed in recent research and policy discussions is the importance of *some kind of informal support network*' (1982:488, emphasis in original).

This perspective also draws attention to the nature and degree of gender-segregation of marital roles, an issue of increasing interest in view of the changing status of women in post-war Britain, which has been one of the most profound social changes of the period. Although many legal and administrative anomalies persist, there has been a substantial catalogue of legislation reflecting, at least in principle, the fact that 'Women now have a status more nearly equivalent to men' (Nissel 1982:110). The way in which couples evolve their role responsibilities, therefore, and the extent to which the marital relationship and roles are segregated – as in the traditional marriage, as opposed to joint, a comparatively recent arrangement thought to be indicative of the modern companionate marriage – has been the subject of substantial research and discussion. As Chester comments:

> 'it would be foolish to doubt that change has occurred in family relationships and in the balance of family types over the past few decades, or that much of this has concerned egalitariansim, de-segregation of roles and partnership.'   (1980:141)

On the other hand, Oakley (1982) argues that the supposed widespread desegregation of gender roles in modern marriages is something of a myth that does not match with the persistence of the conventional family in reality (see also Morris 1985).

Stuckert has indicated that

> 'The roles of husband and wife, like any set of culturally related roles, carry a complex pattern of expectations of the responses which are to come from the other. . . . If these role concepts are similar, communication is easier and relationship between the marriage partners is more satisfactory to both.'
>
> (1973:377)

If husband and wife have different expectations and perceptions of their spouse's role performance, marital happiness may be fundamentally affected. From the practitioner's point of view, the central issue is not whether role patterns are changing or not, but whether the pattern adopted or emerging in a particular marriage is acceptable to both husband and wife, and whether expectations are shared or not. This will determine whether problems will occur for the couple. To complicate matters further, 'increasingly couples must improvise and negotiate a relationship which suits their needs and expectations' (Chester 1980:142), since culturally prescribed patterns are increasingly being challenged. Awareness of role patterns within marriage can therefore be a useful perspective for the social worker (Keily 1984), not least because incompatibility in role expectations may well indicate conflict in other aspects of the relationship and thus possibly a high level of dissatisfaction with the marriage.

In addition, role strain – i.e. stress that a person experiences when they cannot, or find it difficult to, meet the expectations and demands of a role, or set of roles, which may have been initially successfully negotiated – may also be an important source of conflict. Even if only one partner experiences role strain at different points in the marriage, the other might also experience stress when their partner fails to meet these role expectations; and the possibility of both partners simultaneously experiencing role strain, perhaps in their roles as parents, creates considerable potential for conflict and unhappiness. Thus, as we argued earlier, it may be role strain that causes the variations in marital satisfaction at different stages of the family life cycle rather than the passage of time and associated events *per se*.

The changing status of women in society also highlights another important structural issue, for with greater equality comes greater power. The economic dependence of married women on their husbands has long been a major point of attack for critics of marriage, because of its importance in allegedly rendering women comparatively powerless in the marital relationship and confining them to traditional, gender-specific domestic roles. Research in this area has concentrated mainly on the wife's perceptions of the power structure within marriage, and conclusions such as Gillespie's, that 'Husbands gain power in marriage as a class, not as individuals' (1971:445), suggesting that power distribution in marriage is determined solely by external, structural factors, reflect the ideological element implicit in much of the debate. As Safilios-Rothschild (1970) suggests in a review of research into family power structure, however, the situation is much more complex, both methodologically and in reality, than such a simple structural analysis would suggest. Theories about power structure are unlikely to become more sophisticated and valid until they can take account not only of the contributions of a whole range of family members to the balance of power within the family and the marriage, but also of the underlying differences in the degree of affective involvement of one family member with another. Factors such as these determine the balance of power just as much as the degree of economic dependence or otherwise.

This rejection of a crude structural analysis of power and authority within marriage is taken further by Mount:

> 'Intimacy always entails personal authority. In a truly intimate relationship one person makes unique claims upon another . . . the authority is both *partial* and *reciprocal* . . . in this sense [it] does not depend upon inequality . . . it depends solely upon one person acknowledging another person's right to make claims on him.'
>
> (1982:195)

An appreciation of the reciprocal and dynamic qualities of the marital relationship, such as this, makes it clear that even modern companionate marriages, with symmetrical relationships and joint roles, include this element of authority, which critics of marriage and the family so frequently overlook or confuse with power and domination, usually by the husband. It also makes clear the sterile nature of most purely structural analyses of human relationships.

Economic issues

Researchers in Britain have in general paid little attention to the interrelationship of employment and marriage (Chester 1980:109), or even to the particular phenomenon of the working wife. This is perhaps surprising in view of the scale of the changes involved and their supposed impact on married and family life. As Rimmer and Popay note, 'In 1921 less than 10% of married women were in the formal labour force. But . . . by 1979 nearly half of all married women were economically active' (1982:14). Blood (1965) concluded that employment emancipates women from domestication, affecting the power structure in the family by equalizing the relative power of husband and wife; this results in corresponding changes in the division of family labour with the roles of men and women, adults and children, tending to converge and become less segregated. Weller (1968) and King, McIntyre, and Axelson (1968) reached similar conclusions. Burke and Weir (1976), in a study of professional couples, noted that women tended to respond positively to being employed and their husbands to respond negatively. Hicks and Platt (1970) suggest that, where the wife is employed outside the home because of economic pressures rather than by choice, both partners experience a lower degree of marital happiness.

Wright (1978), however, argues that no clear distinctions between the happiness of working and non-working wives can be drawn. Working outside the home and full-time housewifery both have their own costs and benefits attached to them. He concludes:

'in the aggregate "homemakers" are just as happy as women who work and . . . little purpose is served in denying it . . . . Without some appreciation of the outlook and satisfactions of *both* groups, the scholarly study of women will continue to be distracted by a new set of stereotypes that differ in content but not in function from those which have, only recently, been dismantled.'   (Wright 1978:312-13)

Similarly Locksley (1980) concludes that the findings of British research into the impact of wives' working on marital satisfaction are discrepant and therefore inconclusive, although it is obviously a factor that *may* have an impact upon marital satisfaction and family life.

The broader issue of the impact of employment and unemployment on marital happiness and family life is also one that cannot be overlooked. (For a fuller discussion see, for example, Fogarty, Rapoport, and Rapoport 1971, Morris 1985, Moss and Fonda 1980.) 'Work and marriage are the twin drives in the lives of most individuals, particularly men' (Heisler 1984:6), although the demands of both can sometimes conflict. This view is echoed by Chester (1980), who argues that for some sectors of the population – e.g. long-distance lorry drivers, oil-rig workers, seamen, junior hospital doctors in residence, business executives, or salesmen – there is considerable conflict between the demands of occupational involvement and of full participation in home and family life. The extent to which this is seen as problematic will depend substantially upon the wife's attitude to her husband's occupational dedication, whilst we can only speculate about the impact of occupational idiosyncrasies such as shift-work on marital relationships, since these have not been studied in Britain.

In addition, research (e.g. Thornes and Collard 1979) suggests that economic deficiencies of the husband are related to marital instability. Although there are regional variations, unemployment rates are now higher than at any time in the post-war period; as Rimmer and Popay (1982) have argued, of particular concern is the marked increase in the numbers of long-term unemployed. Whilst over three million workers may be registered as out of work, there may be two of three times as many people in families who are experiencing unemployment, since it affects not just the individuals directly concerned but also their families. There is a growing acceptance that unemployment on this scale is likely to continue for some considerable time. Furthermore, the increasing problem of youth unemployment may well result in a delay in young adults leaving their parental homes, at a point in the family life cycle at which evidence suggests marital satisfaction is often at its lowest. It has been suggested that some 68 per cent of under-eighteen-year-olds leaving full-time education will be unable to find work, a figure that is also unlikely to change in the near future (Rimmer and Popay 1982). The Study Commission on the Family comments on this bleak picture:

'The unemployment of young workers may harm family relationships . . . involuntary unemployment will certainly increase in the immediate future causing greater insecurity for families out of work or on the margin of the labour force. Such insecurity can have severe consequences for members of the family including physical, psychological and social disability and maladaption.' (1980:27)

Financial difficulties are frequently associated with unemployment, marginal employment, and marital problems. Smee and Stern have argued that, in spite of the increase in the number of working wives,

'the average family suffering unemployment is not cushioned by the earnings of secondary workers (or at least wives) to anything like the extent suggested by the high incidence of secondary workers in the economy as a whole. The cushion is particularly thin for the families of unemployed unskilled workers, especially those with three or more children.' (1978:10)

Wage levels for many, too, are still woefully inadequate (Rimmer and Popay 1982), and family poverty remains a major problem in Britain – as is apparent from the fact that in March 1981 nearly half of the 103,000 familes drawing Family Income Supplement were two-parent families.

The significance of work in our society is not solely that it generates income, but that it also offers status, identity, interest and companionship. Thus the impact of unemployment can be profound (see, for example, Fagin and Little 1984), research suggesting that 'unemployment is associated with an increased risk of ill-health, emotional disturbance and family breakdown' (Rimmer and Popay 1982:79; see also Rapoport 1981). Unemployment has also been found to be associated variously with vulnerability to psychiatric disorder, levels of hostility amongst out-of-work school-leavers, increased incidence of physical symptoms related to stress, behavioural disorders and poor educational attainment amongst the children of unemployed parents, child abuse, and even admissions of children into care. It may also be, however, that the nature of family and marital relationships is one of the most important factors militating against the worst consequences of unemployment. As Chester concludes,

'there are manifold relationships between class, occupation and work on the one hand and marriage and its problems on the other, even if the relationships are not always well documented or well understood.'   (1980:170)

Sexual problems

The potential for sexual problems at various stages of married life has already been referred to (see pp. 33–39), and it may be helpful to comment on this in more detail outside the framework of the family life cycle. Many such problems are a product of the interaction of individual personality and external factors, especially the marital relationship, and thus are commonly referred to as psychosexual problems, since they are not related solely to sexuality and physiologically based sexual disorders.

Two important perspectives need to be considered. First, there is little research evidence relating to sexual difficulties as marital problems *per se*. In Dominian's (1968) view sexual problems that arise in an otherwise harmonious relationship tend to occur largely because of ignorance of anatomy or technique, or because of environmental pressures of various sorts; 'There are very few marriages in serious difficulty without sexual problems' (Dominian 1968:76). Thus if the main goals of a marital relationship, however a couple may define them, are being achieved, then sexual difficulties can be viewed within a context of overall satisfaction. If there are major relationship difficulties, on the other hand, minor sexual problems may well cause added anxiety, frustrations, and tensions. The result may be that the sexual problem becomes a vehicle used, either consciously or unconsciously, to symbolize all the other difficulties, a definitive statement of dissatisfaction and incompatibility.

The second perspective requires that sexual relationships in modern marriages are put in their social context. One important advance that has stemmed from the emergence of the 'permissive' society has been the liberation of many people from the negative, inhibiting, and even guilt-ridden attitudes that were the legacy of supposed Victorian morality and have, in the past, underpinned some problems of sexual adjustment. But another result has been the raising of much higher expectations of sexual fulfilment, particularly amongst women (see, for example, Gorer 1971:113–29, Chester and Walker 1978), creating another set of problems. Thus the modern ideal of romantic love combined with sexual fulfilment in marriage, in conjunction with other changes already referred to, has created a unique and multi-faceted double-bind:

> 'if two people in a marriage instead of one demand, and have the power to insist on, personal happiness and satisfaction, then clearly the chances of marriages breaking are doubled – probably more than doubled.'   (Gathorne-Hardy 1981:20)

Although sexual problems may be more prevalent at certain stages in married life, the existence of a whole range of pressures, both internal and external to the marriage, may lead to psychosexual problems at any stage; these may in turn contribute to reduced levels of marital satisfaction. Such an understanding may well be essential in achieving a full appreciation of the nature of the problems and behaviours being considered, regardless of whether or not they become the focus for intervention.

Step-families

In our discussion of the family life cycle it was recognized that the increasing numbers of marriages ending in divorce and leading to remarriage do not fit readily into such a framework, experiencing as they do partial and disrupted marital and family development. Whilst many of the comments in the preceding sections are of relevance to remarriages and step-families, they also have many unique features meriting special consideration. For many remarried couples, the former marriage will continue to exert an influence through the existence of children and through the pressures that may be created by both access and the payment of maintenance (see, for example, Burgogyne and Clark 1982b). Wallerstein and Kelly (1980) suggest that, when good ties are maintained by the custodial parent with the non-custodial parent, satisfactory relationships between children and step-parents are more likely, and the pressures therefore are less likely to be problematic. Several studies have referred to the problems of maintaining access to children after divorce, however, and to the general decline in access over time (Eekelaar and Clive 1977, George and Wilding 1972, James and Wilson 1984c, Marsden 1973); also to the conflict and problems often surrounding access and the behavioural disturbances that may be associated with these in some children (Benedek and Benedek 1977, Eekelaar 1982, James and Wilson 1984c, Kelly and Wallerstein 1977, Murch 1980), which may well create tensions and problems for remarried couples.

Thus for those couples who came together to create step-families, many unique and complex problems have to be faced that will exert powerful pressures on the couple and may reduce marital satisfaction. Early studies (e.g. Bowerman and Irish 1962) found some evidence of higher levels of stress in step-families, and the difficult roles of step-parents and in particular stepmothers (witness the extensive mythology of the wicked stepmother) have been widely discussed (Podolsky 1955, Schulman 1972, Visher and Visher 1978a). Recent research (Ferri 1984) confirms the difficult role of stepmother but also its greater potential for success in comparison with the less clear role of stepfather. The stepfather's role may be defined only indirectly, in terms of his relationship with the natural mother, creating the risk that he 'may remain detached from the children with no clearly defined part to play as a source of authority, discipline, advice or affection' (Ferri 1984:118).

Glenn and Weaver (1977) did not find substantial differences in marital happiness between groups of never-divorced and remarried people, however (a view generally endorsed by Albrecht 1979), and suggested that those remarriages that do not end quickly in divorce are probably as successful as intact first marriages. Spanier and Furstenberg (1982) also concluded that individuals typically appear to fare better when remarriages are successful and rewarding than they would have done if they had remained divorced. They none the less point out that the opposite effect may occur when a remarriage is experienced as unrewarding, in that an individual's sense of initial failure may be reinforced, reducing his or her sense of well-being. Duberman (1973) suggests that the increased complexity of inter- and intra-familial relationships presents many of the problems in step-families, whilst, in addition, all of the normal problems existing between siblings also exist in step-families in an exaggerated form and

have to be dealt with by the remarried couple. Thus Duberman
concludes that

> 'the reconstituted family must make self-conscious efforts to
> establish itself as an entity . . . the members have separate histories
> and memories; different concepts of roles, values, norms and goals.
> Solidarity, the concept of themselves as a functioning unit, must be
> carefully cultivated if it is to be achieved.'   (1973:291–92)

Visher and Visher (1979) suggest that step-families experience
particular problems in coping with these difficulties. The previous
experience of 'failure' in a former marriage can lead to a denial of the
existence of problems in the remarriage, whilst a lack of understanding and knowledge of the problems of step-parent–stepchild
relationships in particular, and of step-family problems in general,
can inhibit the disclosure of such difficulties to others. Furthermore,
insecurity of either parents or children in their 'step-roles' can inhibit
exploration and resolution of even minor issues that would be unproblematic in biological families. In addition to step-parents often
having unrealistically high expectations of themselves – 'instant love'
of their stepchildren, for example – there may be particular problems
in integrating families containing teenagers, often related to the usual
tensions and pressures as teenaged children grow up and away from
their families. These may be exacerbated by their emerging sexuality,
which may make it difficult for teenagers to deal with 'the sexualized
atmosphere of the stepfamily' (Visher and Visher 1982b), since the
sexuality of recently married adults is much more difficult to ignore or
deny than it is in the biological family, in which parents tend to be
seen by their children as non-sexual beings. Added to this already
complex and potentially difficult situation is the problem for the new
couple of finding the time and the space, both in emotional and perhaps even in physical terms, to nourish and develop their own couple
relationship, which is so essential to the solidarity and stability of the
new marriage and family.

Research in Britain by Burgoyne and Clark (1981, 1982a, 1982b,
1984) confirms many of the findings referred to above. They propose
that the step-family has a life cycle of its own (1982b), whilst others
have also attempted to identify the developmental stages that are
unique to step-family formation (see, for example, Ransom, Schlesinger, and Derdeyn 1979). However, Burgoyne and Clark (1981) also
point out the dangers associated with ascribing too much importance to
the *step*-family as a source of problems; they found that, in many cases,

the problems experienced by step-parents seemed very similar to those experienced by parents in first marriages.

Step-families do have some unique problems with which to contend. These are in part derived from the predominant ideal of the conventional nuclear family in modern Britain and the consequent 'marginality' of the step-family, which is reflected in the ambiguity of the step-relationship in the eyes of the law (Parry 1983). Importantly, however, Ferri concludes that

> 'it remains true that the majority of children, even in stepfather families, seemed to enjoy satisfactory home relationships, to be making similar educational progress to children in other situations and to hold equally positive aspirations for their own future.'
>
> (1984:116–17)

Besides the research referred to in this section, there is a growing list of publications through which we can seek to increase our understanding of the step-family (see, for example, Brown 1982, Furstenberg and Spanier 1984, Robinson 1980, Walker *et al.* 1979), as well as to explore ways in which appropriate help might be made available to them (Burgoyne 1984, Johnson 1980, Messinger 1976, Pill 1981, Visher and Visher 1978b, 1982a). The social worker must be aware not only of the potential for difficulties in such family situations, but also the many pressures against the disclosure of any such difficulties to helping agencies. The possibility of similar or related problems for adoptive or foster-parents should also be borne in mind.

Ethnicity

Britain is a multi-racial society in which about three million immigrants and their descendants live, about half of whom are whites from Ireland, Europe, and the Old Commonwealth, the other half being non-whites mainly from the New Commonwealth countries of Asia, Africa, and the West Indies. Ethnic minorities tend to be geographically concentrated in areas such as Greater London, Birmingham, and Bradford. In 1977, for example, 4 per cent of the population of Greater London was of West Indian origin and 4 per cent of Asian origin; in Birmingham 5 per cent were West Indian and 6 per cent Asian; whilst in Bradford less than 1 per cent were West Indian, and 8 per cent were Asian (Eversley and Bonnerjea 1982; see also British Association of Social Workers 1982). The term 'Asian' is an imprecise one; it groups Punjabis, Tamils, Pakistanis, and Bangladeshis together in a way that, whilst generally useful in a descriptive sense, conceals as many cultural differences as it suggests similarities (see Ballard 1982, Kinnon 1984).

It is appropriate to give particular attention to the question of marital problems amongst ethnic minorities. We must question the relevance of the preceding discussion to ethnic minorities because, as Chester (1980) has pointed out, researchers in the field of marital problems have given little attention to the issue of ethnicity. There is little ethnic-related statistical information about even such basic facts as rates of marriage and marriage breakdown, because of the sensitive issue of gathering ethnically specific data. It would be dangerous to assume that marriage is either more or less popular, or marriage breakdown is either more or less common, amongst ethnic minorities (although some observers believe it is increasing – see Blair *et al.* 1981); or that it is necessarily influenced in the same way by the many social, economic, and psychological factors referred to in preceding sections of this chapter.

We do know, however, that in comparison with the indigenous population, the New Commonwealth and Pakistani populations are comparatively young, reflecting not only the demographic character-istics of many immigrants but also the fact that much immigration has been comparatively recent. We also know that unemployment amongst ethnic minorities has remained consistently higher and has increased proportionately more quickly than amongst the population as a whole (Smith 1976, 1981). Many ethnic minority groups have been forced to settle in the decaying inner and middle rings of large cities, find it harder than whites to rent accommodation or to buy houses (Foner 1977, Runnymede Trust 1980), and are more likely to be generally disadvantaged (Osborn, Butler, and Morris 1984). Marriage and family patterns tend to differ historically amongst ethnic minority groups, and different groups have been influenced to varying degrees by British cultural patterns. Triseliotis (1972) points out, for example, that Indian and Pakistani families are closely knit and cohesive, in marked contrast to the looser and more open West Indian family; and whilst the semi-extended West Indian and Cypriot family group can tolerate a degree of disagreement and internal conflict, the more closely knit Indian and Pakistani families, in which dissension and conflict are neither encouraged nor tolerated, will not openly admit to internal conflict and disagreements.

Foner believes that Jamaicans have been influenced by the norms of English family life, and that these changes are due to the absence of kin in England, 'combined with a normative stress on the desirability of joint husband–wife activities in England . . . wives tend to look to their spouses for some of the comfort and companionship they formerly found with relatives.'   (1977:142)

Khan (1977) and Catherine Ballard (1979) have noted, in contrast, the persistence of Asian family structures, values, and institutions. As Catherine Ballard has pointed out, this has important implications, since whilst many second-generation Asians do rebel against parental values and controls in their teens (in which respect they are not unlike their white counterparts), resulting in clashes and disruptions in the family, by their late teens and early twenties the majority of them substantially accept and conform to Asian norms within the sphere of life in the family and the community – a view supported by Weinreich (1979).

The traditional Asian (and Cypriot) concept of marriage is based on the choice of a suitable partner by the parents. Love, so central to the formation of marriages in British society, is expected to come after the marriage and not before. Many young Asians, although they approach such marriages with trepidation, accept arranged marriages (Ahmed 1981), and this is made easier for many by the possibility of exercising some covert and discreet influence on the choice of their parents. Having done so, many couples find that they do achieve a satisfactory relationship, which often begins to develop to some extent along non-traditional lines, with less formal and more egalitarian relations, more shared and companionate activities and more importance being attached to their separate identities. The birth of the first child may be postponed to give them more time to become acquainted and more freedom, with social networks being developed on the basis of interest and compatibility in contrast to the kin-dominated world of their parents. Many Asians, including many of the second generation, would maintain, according to Catherine Ballard (1979), that such arranged marriages are based on sounder foundations than 'love marriages' and that they are probably less likely to fail (see also Marett 1983).

Such marriages do sometimes fail nevertheless, for a variety of reasons. Ballard and Ballard (1977) have suggested that it may be increasingly difficult, for example, for parents to make a good choice of partner in a context of rapid social change and of both generation and culture gaps between parents and children; parents of peasant origin may have highly educated children, and the negotiations are now sometimes entrusted to an intermediary rather than being conducted directly by the family themselves. Sanctions that were traditionally

available in relation to marital disputes and problems may be ineffective in a British context, whilst the fragmentation of the extended
family, which has occurred for many, may put much greater strain on
the marital relationship, a view echoed by Khan (1977) and Rack
(1979). Similarly, some new brides, brought up within the context of
their traditional extended family at home, may find themselves coming
to a situation for which they are unprepared, where they are living with
their husbands alone. Even where there is mutual affection and
kindness, the emotional intensity engendered by such a situation may
be difficult to cope with. Rack suggests that, as a result,

> 'There are some unfortunate Pakistani girls in England, whose
> marriages are unhappy, who are completely at the mercy of their
> husbands because they have no other relatives in this country'.
>
> (1979:178–79)

Other researchers have drawn attention to significant differences in
cultural background and expectations for other ethnic minorities, such
as West Africans (Goody and Groothues 1977, 1979), Cypriots (Oakley
1982), and the Chinese (Watson 1977), but there is still no clear picture
of the nature, incidence, and distribution of marital problems. As
Cheetham (1981) has argued, most social work contacts with members
of ethnic minority groups tend to be confined to intervention in fairly
dramatic examples of family conflict and stress. Social workers too
often regard the cultural differences that may seem to underlie some of
these problems as disadvantages, giving too little attention to the
advantages and benefits that also exist and the strengths they contain
whereby many individuals are helped to cope with their problems. It is
also important, however, not to become over-reliant upon a cultural
frame of reference that may distract attention not only from significant
emotional factors, but also from structural factors such as class, race,
and economic pressures (Ahmed 1983). As Ballard and Ballard have
commented, 'It is clear that any understanding of racial and ethnic
minorities must rest on a consideration of both the internal preferences
and the external constraints which act simultaneously upon them'
(1977:53–4). This succinctly summarizes the challenge presented to
social workers of understanding marital problems amongst ethnic
minorities.

Problems for social work agencies

The foregoing pages have offered an outline of some of the many different problems with which married couples may have to cope at various points in their life together, and which may lead to attempts to seek help, whether or not the problem is actually defined as a marital problem. Brannen and Collard (1982) draw attention to the distinction between those who define their marriages as problematic and those where the agency makes the definition. In the former, the spouses had usually experienced a marital problem or even a crisis, and many such couples will approach specialized marriage-guidance agencies. In the latter group, however, the decision to seek help was usually preceded by an individual crisis. The conflicting pressures for couples in such situations are summed up by Brannen and Collard thus:

> 'avoiding the definition of marital problems may sustain the marriage but it often seemed to do so at the expense of the health of at least one of the partners. On the other hand, defining a marital problem is inherently a risky business, since it . . . may ultimately lead to the breakup of the marriage.'   (1982:111)

As *Marriage Matters* (Home Office 1979) observed, therefore, it is perhaps not surprising that many people with marriage-related difficulties should seek help from a range of agencies not specifically concerned or identified with marital problems.

The largest of these are, of course, social services departments. Whilst they have no statutory duty to undertake marital counselling, they do have a responsibility to undertake work with a range of family problems. Many of their clients may have marital problems that are presented covertly through apparently unrelated problems to do with health, housing, finance, or child care (*Marriage Matters*, Home Office 1979, Tebboth 1981). Mattinson and Sinclair (1979) found that the large majority of the cases that social workers regarded as the most demanding and the highest priority involved marital problems, although this did not necessarily mean that any marital work was being attempted with them. Although the possible significance of organizational factors in this should not be overlooked, *Marriage Matters* refers to 'some resistance, particularly among younger social workers, to "probing" into personal problems particularly if these are not the direct presenting problem' (Home Office 1979:140). Also, as Mattinson and Sinclair remark, whilst 'it is certainly possible to do marital work in a social services department . . . for the inexperienced social worker, unsure of his own skill, it is certainly easier to avoid it' (1979:289).

Social workers must therefore be sensitive to the possibility of marital problems when dealing with a wide range of referrals. Parents of handicapped children, for example, experience not only additional stresses in parenting but sometimes feelings of guilt and fear of further pregnancies, which may in turn lead to sexual problems (Kew 1974). The death of a child in a family can also precipitate a marital crisis (Craig 1974). Married couples who are themselves handicapped are likely to experience particular difficulties, and there are now a large number of elderly married couples who may be encountering marital problems resulting from changed physical, emotional, economic, and social circumstances, whose difficulties may not be recognized, assessed, or dealt with (Bull 1984). The problems of marital work with ethnic minorities have also been referred to (see pp. 49–52), although in a recent survey of social services and ethnic minorities (Association of Directors of Social Services 1983) this particular issue receives no mention. As Bull has argued, our 'assumptions and presumptions about the needs of particular "client groups" are due for re-examination' (1984:56), particularly with regard to the existence of and possibilities for intervention in marital problems.

There are also clear links between marital problems and health. Renne (1971) found that physical and psychological health was related to marital happiness; Brown and Harris (1978) suggested that the quality of the marital relationship was one of the principal factors putting women at risk from depression following a severe life event; Hooper, Hinchcliff, and Roberts (1978) explored the interrelationship between marriage and depression in a broader context; and, as the Royal College of General Practitioners comments in its evidence in *Marriage Matters*, 'Marital unhappiness can present as depression, as a headache or a backache or a heavy period or a child who refuses to go to school' (Home Office 1979:145). 'What can safely be concluded is that sometimes there is a medical dimension to troubled marriage' (Chester 1980:212), a fact of which all helping professionals in medical settings should be aware.

In contrast, the probation service has a long-standing involvement in work with marital problems and a statutory involvement with the domestic courts dating back to 1937. Whilst there has been a decline in matrimonial referrals in recent years, partly because of the growth of alternative sources of help and of easier and cheaper divorce, the association between crime, marital tensions, and marital breakdown is a well-established one (see, for example, Rutter and Giller 1983, West 1982). Although marital problems are not invariably associated with criminal behaviour, they are directly or indirectly important in many cases involving both adults and juveniles, and a central factor in some. Evidence from the probation service in *Marriage Matters* also indicates, however, that

> 'There is a certain amount of collusion by probation officers in the diminution of marital work. Young officers lack the self-confidence to help and are increasingly reluctant to undertake marital work, and this is mainly due to lack of adequate training.'
>
> (Home Office 1979:137)

It is also worth referring to the relationship between alcoholism and marital problems, both general and sexual. The association between alcohol and a range of social problems is well documented, but the focus is less often upon the marital problems that may be one of either the causes or the effects of alcohol abuse. Problem drinking can constitute a major source of stress for marriages and families (see, for example, Camberwell Council on Alcoholism 1980, Edwards 1982, Grant and Gwinner 1979, Hunt 1982, Krasner, Madden, and Walker 1984, Orford and Harwin 1982, Royal College of Psychiatrists 1979), and there are also links between alcohol and violence both within and without marriages (Chester 1980), which may also present an opportunity for social-work intervention.

It is perhaps not surprising to find that the potential for marital problems exists alongside so many of the problems encountered by social workers. A major difficulty for social work agencies, however, is not only that of seeing through the presenting problems (many of which will of course be very real) to the underlying emotional problems with which they will frequently be associated, but also encouraging amongst social workers the willingness to do this and to take the lid off this daunting Pandora's box.

Homeostasis in marital relationships

The preceding pages of this chapter have been devoted almost exclusively to evidence concerning problems in marital relationships, but it is important to remember that the majority of marriages remain intact. Few attempts have been made to study the factors that, in spite of the endless assault of difficulties with which they must contend, enable many couples to cope with and rise above the adversity that may at times seem virtually to besiege them and their families. As Gathorne-Hardy has eloquently expressed it,

> 'Happy families may resemble each other, but each marriage at the centre of that family is happy in its own particular way. The ties

that bind people, the needs they fulfil in each other, are as complex or simple, as deep or shallow, often as unknowable as the people themselves . . . . And this is still more complicated because we are always both in the stream of becoming, while all the time wanting to be fixed.'   (1981:158)

The same paradox was recently explored by Askham (1984). The more that basic economic and material needs are satisfied, the more central personal growth becomes to the relationship, which requires us to recognize the importance of historical continuity in marriages, for 'Marriage is the place where the past is most active in the present' (Gathorne-Hardy 1981:262). This perspective is, as we shall later argue, of particular importance in relation to some explanations of marital behaviour. Its immediate significance is that it reflects the dynamic nature of the marital relationship and the forces that keep it intact.

An important attempt to conceptualize this was made by Levinger (1965), who outlined a framework that attempted to integrate the conflicting forces, some of which hold a couple together whilst others threaten to pull them apart, which is not without empirical support (Udry 1981). This encompassed the satisfactions and attractions of the marriage, and the negative unsatisfying aspects; the strength of the inducements to leave the marriage, including the attractiveness of alternatives, as opposed to the strengths of the reasons for staying; and the presence or absence, and relative strengths and weaknesses, of the restraints against breaking up the relationship. Hart (1976) proposed a similar model for marital *breakdown*, which focusses attention upon those factors tending to reduce the level of commitment or the value attached to the marital relationship, those factors tending to worsen conflict between the couple or to reduce their ability to cope with tension, and those factors that increase the opportunities for individuals to escape from their marriages.

The attractiveness of these approaches lies in their ability to encompass the entire range of factors both external and internal to marriage and the family. They can also suggest possible points of focus for intervention, e.g. increasing the relationship's positive attractiveness, decreasing the attractiveness of alternative relationships or circumstances, or increasing the strength of the barriers against marital breakdown. As Levinger (1976) later argued, the private lives of marriage partners are inseparable from events in the social and economic environment in which the marriage exists, and factors both internal and external to the relationship can influence its dissolution or its survival:

'Although it spotlights the dyad, this perspective does not intend that the pair be seen as a closed system. Both cultural norms and social networks have important effects, which can be translated into forces of attraction or restraint.'   (Levinger 1976:44)

A common theme implicit in much of the literature is the central importance of effective communication between partners, an issue explicitly addressed by authors such as Noller (1984). Thornes and Collard (1979) suggest that effective communication requires the opportunity to communicate – in terms both of physical presence and the willingness to disclose or recognize needs and expectations, as well as of a willingness to meet the needs and expectations of the other. This may be more important to women than to men. Klemer (1970) has also stressed the importance of sexual communication in marriage, not just as a means of resolving problems but as a potential source of enrichment for the relationship. Thornes and Collard conclude that effective communication has

'increasing relevance to marital stability as opposed simply to marital happiness . . . if mutual needs are to be adequately recognised, understood and satisfied, effective communication between partners seems essential, otherwise marital dissolution may result since the barriers to divorce have diminished and there now exist more options to remaining in an unhappy marriage.'   (1979:139)

Summary

In this chapter we have offered an analysis of the many and varied problems with which married couples may have to contend, and a review of some of the evidence about marital problems and their sometimes unclear relationship with happiness and satisfaction. The marital relationship tends to be romanticized and idealized, invested with high expectations of love and happiness, security, status, and companionship within a stable relationship. As Belshaw and Strutt amongst others (e.g. Askham 1984) have pointed out, however,

'These powerful ideas which in some measure cater for important needs may, at the same time, cut across the unconscious yet vital needs of two individuals; the psychological and almost biological urge to change and develop throughout adult life. The maturing has to continue during a close relationship such as marriage; indeed it is a function of it.'   (1984:43)

Thus, a marriage must contend with stresses and strains both from within and without, and must be able to adapt if it is not to crumble.

The evidence reviewed suggests that many of these problems may, directly or indirectly, result in a situation that might lead to the involvement of any one of a number of social work agencies, although those that do not specialize in working with marital problems may well not identify, let alone work with, underlying problems of this sort. We have argued that there is enormous scope for such involvement. As Bull has concluded,

> 'There is a need for the early recognition of marital difficulties and for help with them . . . throughout the life-cycle at potential crisis points from ante-natal clinic attendance and before to Pre-Retirement Association advice and guidance and beyond.'   (1984:54)

There is, however, a danger that marital problems might come to be viewed as the subject of yet another specialism along with areas such as problem drinking, drug abuse, and child abuse, which requires such problems to be referred on to a specialist worker or agency. We believe, on the contrary, that intervention with marital problems is within the competence of all trained social workers. As *Marriage Matters* (Home Office 1979) argues, 'the agency of first approach may be the one which can, in many cases, be in a position to provide the best help' (para. 4.88, 53).

The almost overwhelming range of potential problems and difficulties that have been identified is such as to raise the question of why even more marriages do not end in divorce, and yet this is the outcome for only the minority. Regardless of the social construction and definition of marital problems, it is ultimately the behaviour of the spouses towards each other that is of first importance in assessing the existence or otherwise of a marital problem and, crucially, their perception of this. This is not to suggest that only when clients identify themselves as having marital problems does a social worker begin to think of working with these; but the impact of these various pressures and problems on marriage is not universal, and particular problems encountered by social workers must be approached with a keen awareness of their uniqueness within the context of an individual marriage:

> 'Marriage, love relationships, are above all about feelings and emotions. An analysis of great social movements, however profound, and however illuminating, does not seem quite real.'
>
> (Gathorne-Hardy 1981:266)

The task lying before us is to explore some of the ways social workers can begin to analyse and understand these uniquely complex marital relationships, and to make their own unique helping contribution when the opportunity arises.

3

Explanatory concepts

Three principal theoretical approaches have influenced the development and practice of marital therapy in Britain and the United States: psychodynamic, systems, and behavioural theory. Of the three, only the first has been applied with any consistency in Britain to marital problems, through the writings of the Institute of Marital Studies. Consequently, this is the approach with which British social workers are most familiar, although apart from Dicks's (1967) work their writings are hardly known in the United States. It has tended, perhaps unfortunately, to dwarf the contributions of other approaches, which may in fact be more easily understood and used by social workers in non-specialist settings.

Workers in Britain, by tradition and perhaps inclination, draw selectively on theory rather than sticking rigidly to one conceptual approach to intervention. There may therefore be some disadvantages in considering the theoretical formulations of these approaches separately, but we have adopted this format because we believe the ideas may be easier to grasp when presented in this way. What follows is a discussion of the basic concepts of each approach in their application to marital problems, concluding with a summary of those ideas that we consider most relevant to work in this area.

Psychodynamic approaches

Erikson (1965), in his discussion of the interactive and opposing forces operating in emotional development, describes the emotional task of marriage as Intimacy versus Isolation. This graphic description serves as a useful starting point to our discussion since it implicitly highlights two concepts that are central to the psychodynamic approach to marital problems: first, the idea of the 'self' as a central organizing core of the personality, which needs to achieve mastery of certain tasks in order to function satisfactorily; and second, the idea of marriage as functional – i.e. fulfilling a purpose in terms of the needs of the individuals concerned.

Erikson's view of personality development is rooted in object relations theory, and it is this particular psychoanalytic school of thought that has, in our view, contributed most to the understanding and treatment of marital discord. The contributions of writers in the psychoanalytic field outside the 'British School' are not discussed here, since they seem to have less to offer social-work practitioners.

The difference between classical Freudian theory and object relations theory lies chiefly in the shift away from an emphasis on instinctive drives and their neurotic derivations, to the study of the development of the personality in the context of interpersonal relationships. This shift essentially paved the way for, among other things, Bowlby's important work on attachment, separation, and loss (Bowlby 1971). The view of the personality as one in which the need for a satisfying object relationship constitutes the fundamental motive for life was developed by Fairbairn in a seminal work published in 1954. It stresses the simultaneous build-up of the self and of object representation or 'internal objects' – 'object' being a general term for a source of satisfaction of needs that may not always be a person. The self is seen as a composite structure derived from the integration of multiple self-images. In the same way the 'internal objects' are derived from the gradual integration of multiple object-images into comprehensive representations of others. Thus the psychologically healthy individual is one whose cohesive, well-integrated sense of self is balanced by realistic, well-differentiated images of others.

A child's relationship with its primary caretakers in its early years is held to be crucially important to the development of personality. Bowlby, from observation of the behaviour of young children and primates, developed the idea of a process of attachment, through which a bond between mother-figure and child is established. Defining attachment behaviour as 'seeking and maintaining proximity to another individual' (Bowlby 1971:241), he argued that it is biologically based and is displayed most readily between the ages of 7 months and 3 years, although it can be elicited at any age. Some of Bowlby's original formulations concerning attachment behaviour have attracted widespread criticism (e.g. Schaffer 1971); but it may be accepted, as Rutter argues, that attachment is 'a fundamental characteristic of the mother–child relationship' (1981:14).

Other key concepts of object relations theory concern the mechanisms by which the developing personality gradually becomes able to hold on to the knowledge of the attachment figure as dependable and loving, even in the absence of that figure or in the midst of frustration. When a child experiences frustration, this arouses a sense of conflict between his experience and need to perceive the attachment figure as good and loving, and his experience of her as bad or rejecting. The theory suggests that this threat to the structure of self is dealt with by the defence mechanism known as splitting, so that one part of the good object, stripped of its distressing characteristics, can remain as a satisfying memory, whilst negative aspects are repressed. Although thus repressed, these psychological systems remain within the personality structure, seeking a resolution of the conflict that generated them. This process of introjection, splitting, repression, and resolution-seeking is seen as a normal part of development. Where the personality is reasonably secure and resilient, and the need to split and repress is not overwhelming because the conflict between good and bad is not extreme, many of these split-off systems may be reintegrated. Alternatively, the earlier in life at which splitting occurs and the more distressing and frustrating the experience of the external object world, the greater will be the intensity of the splitting and the power and dependence on the inner world. Thus, whether the painful experience remains split off and repressed, or is retested and reintegrated into the central ego, depends on both the intensity and degree of repression, and the extent to which subsequent relations with the intimate other tend to confirm or disprove the child's fear.

As we suggest below, there are a number of criticisms to be levelled at object relations theory, not least amongst which is the difficulty of defining the concepts with precision, thus making the merits of the various hypotheses often impossible to test and establish. None the less, as Segraves argues, it does provide the practitioner with a useful organizing framework that 'does justice to the complexity of the nuances of human behaviour in intimate relationships' (1982:71), and as we argue later, some of these concepts are useful to practitioners even if the higher-level abstractions of the theory remain questionable (see, for example, Segraves 1982 and Gurman 1978 for a fuller discussion of these issues).

APPLICATION TO MARITAL INTERACTION

A detailed application of the concepts of object relations to marital interaction is to be found in the writings of the Institute of Marital Studies (IMS) (e.g. Bannister and Pincus 1965, Mainprice 1974, Pincus 1960). The reader is referred to these for a fuller discussion than is possible here. Their conception of marital interaction is based on the premise that the choice of marital partner is influenced by the unconscious need of the individual to get in touch with split-off and repressed elements of his personality, and that the extent to which the marriage is satisfying or conflict-ridden will depend on the extent to which these needs are fulfilled.

Dicks (1967), in the most coherent if most abstract formulation of these ideas, suggests that there are three major levels that may be involved in the selection of marital partners, which serve to maintain or disrupt the couple's cohesion, and that there must be satisfaction at two levels at least for the marriage to remain viable. The first level is that of socio-cultural values and norms. Although, as we argued in Chapter 1, marriage in Britain has long emphasized the free choice of a partner based on ideas of romantic love and mutual satisfaction of needs, socio-economic factors also exert a powerful influence on choice, producing high levels of homogamy in marriage.

The second level Dicks delineates as that of 'central egos', where the personal norms and values, conscious judgements, beliefs, and expectations are operating in the choice of partner. At this level, the ongoing demands of each partner on the other in their role of husband/wife, partner/lover, etc. continually test the consistency between consciously held attitudes and actual behaviour. Where there is a reasonable degree of integration — i.e. where conscious beliefs and role models are congruent with the individual's internalized world — then there is likely to be a consistency between the couple's initial mutual expectations and their experience of interaction. If, for example, a man's stated rational belief in the equality of women is derived from his early experiences, then it is likely that his behaviour within the marital relationship will be more or less consistent with his rational belief. Where the rational belief conflicts with his internalized world — e.g. if as a child he has experienced a very unequal relationship between his parents — there may be difficulty. The hypothesis would be that, where this facet of the relationship has been introjected with relatively little stress, then this inconsistency between rational behaviour and subconscious expectation or wish may be relatively easily resolved. Dicks points out that it is at this level that such qualities as tolerance and flexibility are important in enabling the couple to adapt to and accept each other's changing needs and developing identity.

Sometimes, however, relationships may end in disarray where the shared beliefs and ideals that have formed the basis of their earlier union have diverged. An example of this may be found in the film *The Way We Were*, in which Robert Redford and Barbra Streisand appear as two students drawn together by an interest in creative writing, who subsequently marry. The hero becomes successful and, his moral and political seriousness dwindling, he can no longer satisfy or gain satisfaction from his wife's more intense nature, and they part, relatively amicably. Dicks argues that this kind of growing apart and altering in more or less conscious interests and attitudes gives rise, in theory at least, to relatively painless and reasoned partings.

At the third and last level, Dicks focusses on the *un*conscious object-relational needs that flow between marriage partners and require satisfaction and feedback:

> 'the partner attracts because he or she represents or promises a re-discovery of an important lost aspect of the subject's own personality, which, owing to earlier conditioning, had been recast as an object for attack or denial.'   (1967:30)

In other words it is argued that very often in marriage, an individual is drawn to another because that other seems able to supply and express certain aspects of personality that the individual has repressed and failed to integrate into his own. In accordance with the proposition of object relations theory that these aspects or systems remain active and seek resolution and integration, the marital choice is therefore also founded on the wish to know more about these disowned parts in order that they should be integrated into the whole. That this process should occur within marriage is explicable if we consider that through physical closeness, loving, and caring it offers people the opportunity to get as close as they are ever likely to get to the feelings they experienced in their very early relationships. It also helps to explain why some form attachments that cause them much distress, whilst others may become professionally successful or socially competent but are unable to tolerate intimacy or make viable lasting relationships (e.g. as in Aldous Huxley's novel *Genius and the Goddess*, 1955).

This hypothesis of complementary needs has gained some support from writers and practitioners outside the IMS. Skynner, for example, states that 'couples are usually attracted by shared developmental failures' (1976:43), and Meissner writes of couples who 'tend to choose partners who have achieved an equivalent level of immaturity' (1978:43). Marriage may therefore be seen as a second chance, offering a couple the opportunity to make good past failures and enabling them to grow and develop. Where the difficulty and failure to integrate have not been acute, the experience of marriage may be satisfying and thera-peutic, particularly where other aspects of the marriage are supportive and comparatively conflict-free. Thus a man who has difficulty in expressing feelings may, by marrying a less inhibited wife, gradually learn to feel comfortable with a greater degree of expressiveness within the context of a secure relationship, so that his own internal prohibi-tions and fears (essentially of the loss of a vital relationship if he behaves expressively) are gradually lifted.

The need-complementarity hypothesis is a complex one, and the reader is referred to Gurman (1978) for a critical evaluation and discus-sion. It is argued, however, that couples who experience difficulties may do so because those very qualities that drew them together are conscious expressions of what, at an unconscious level, they each find difficult. Different behaviours may reflect what is in fact a similar unconscious difficulty; uninhibited behaviour may be a vigorous attempt to deal with exactly the same difficulties of reserve that a partner may respond to in the opposite way.

Since the way this theoretical approach is formulated and the detail is developed is complex, it may be helpful to summarize its key points:

1 Marriage problems are hardly ever 'caused' primarily by one partner or the other. They are almost always the result of collusion, an uncon-scious agreement between the couple. The difficulty is thus usually a shared one; e.g. if one partner is struggling with feelings of sexual coldness, then it is likely that at some level this is a problem for both.
2 The mechanisms of defence that are used to maintain this collusion are principally those of splitting, denial, projection, and projective identification.
3 Where displaced feelings are projected on to the marital partner, then the personality of that partner will almost invariably offer some basis in reality for the projection; one person is unlikely to accept the projections unless at some level there is a 'fit'. The accep-tance of these feelings is called 'introjection'.
4 Frequently, the projection of disowned, repressed wishes and desires on to the other partner leads to that partner having to express what is called a 'double dose' — i.e. their own feelings about, for example,

domination, as well as their partner's. This leads to further unhappiness and friction, since one partner is having to play an exaggerated part in expressing those feelings, whilst the partner who escapes the 'double dose' does so at the expense of failing to experience and integrate their own feelings about dominance and control. Alternatively, the split may occur between the couple and the outside world. Where the relationship is idealized, conflict becomes impermissible, and the external world is 'bad'; or conversely, only negative feelings may be allowed within the dyad, whilst good feelings are projected on to others.

5 Resolving mechanisms are held to be those of recognition and depression followed by integration.

6 The rigidity of a split can be measured by the degree to which mixed feelings towards one another cannot be acknowledged. As Mattinson and Sinclair say, 'there are few greys in the world of the person prone to compulsive splitting; it is seen in extremes of black and white' (1979:55).

7 The difficulties arising from this kind of splitting take different forms, but their origin will be in the discomfort resulting from the continuing struggle with the disowned feelings. Thus, a husband may deal with his anxieties and ambivalence about dominance by putting his wife in the dominant position and maintaining a stance of resentful ineffectualness, whilst his wife may accept the role of capable carer at the cost of having to deny her own feelings of dependency. The very incompleteness of the part each is enacting will lead to continuing anxiety and frustration.

We do not, as Guthrie and Mattinson say in their booklet,

> 'know how people manage to put feelings (which are either appropriate or inappropriate to the situation) . . . out of their own psychological system into that of another person.' (1971:44)

It is nevertheless a process with which we are all to some extent familiar. The concept of scapegoating, where one person is made to carry the sins of the rest, so that the group can continue to deny ownership of these sinful feelings (and therefore escape the risk of their being translated into action similar to that of the person scapegoated), is one well-known manifestation of the mechanism of splitting and projection. Within the couple relationship, as has been suggested, the process may become one of projective identification, so that in the course of trying to repair the split and bring the feelings back into themselves the individual may select a partner who can be the recipient of the feelings. This process of projective identification is not limited to familial relationships, although it is most commonly observed there, but is probably confined to relationships of intimacy, even if these are brief. There is a graphic account of the way splitting and projective identification can occur in Conrad's (1926) short story *The Secret Sharer*,[1] to which the reader is referred for an exposition of what can sometimes seem an elusive and difficult phenomenon.

Our discussion shows that this approach to marital interaction emphasizes those difficulties that have to do with the inter-working of the inner worlds of the individuals – i.e. where there is conflict at Dicks's third level of unconscious needs. This seems to be a major deficiency in the approach, because, as is evident from our experience and from some of the research discussed later, many couples who experience difficulties and seek help with their relationship are not in conflict at this level, although they are experiencing great distress. In addition, little attention is paid to the possibility of working with difficulties that are occurring at a conscious level – e.g. conflict over role expectations and behaviour – even where there are difficulties at an unconscious level that remain untouched. Gurman, comparing contemporary marital therapies, sees the major deficiency in psychoanalytic approaches as the fact that they pay 'insufficient attention to the current and actual sources of interaction that maintain marital conflict beyond the distortions engendered in the marital transference' (1978:456). This is not to say, as one might of the classical psychoanalytic approach, that past childhood experiences (issues concerning infantile impulses and especially separation – individuation) are emphasized at the expense of looking at current interaction; but rather that those aspects of current interaction that reflect unconscious collusion are emphasized at the expense of those that do not, but which may in themselves be contentious.

This weakness has in our view had the damaging effect of making work with marital problems appear esoteric, drawing attention away from the possibilities of alternative ways of intervening. It must be acknowledged that there is no suggestion that the intervention itself must be interpretative, whatever the explanatory framework used by the workers, a fact that Guthrie and Mattinson (1971) for example make quite clear. None the less, there is an implicit suggestion that all marital problems are of a collusive nature and a consequent lack of attention to the possibility of adopting a different emphasis or more limited approach. In addition, it is difficult to extrapolate precepts about intervention in marital problems. All these factors have, in our view, contributed to the tendency amongst social workers to avoid the problems that couples experience with their relationships.

A further criticism, also made by Gurman (1978), is that many of the concepts used in object relations theory have as yet not had empirical validation. As he points out, there has not yet been empirical study of many central psychoanalytic constructs, including collusion, projective identification, marital transference, idealization, fusion, differentiation, and individuation, nor is there any empirical support for some of the central propositions of the theory about marital dynamics. The difficulty of envisaging a feasible way of gaining valid empirical evidence is related to the difficulty referred to earlier of generalizing and utilizing the concepts.

Finally, the focus in the early IMS work on collusive marriages and the defence mechanisms of splitting, projection, and projective identification has led to an under-emphasis on the concept of attachment and attachment behaviour, which is, in our view, of central importance in understanding the needs and behaviour of adults in intimate relationships, compared with other close relationships. Mattinson and Sinclair (1979) remedy this, pointing out that an understanding of attachment behaviour (and how, for example, it becomes more pronounced in times of stress or under threat of loss) was crucial to their understanding of the clients in their study, and that 'Marriage gives the opportunity for reattachment to a specific figure, and legally sanctions attachment behaviour' (Mattinson and Sinclair 1979:49). It is with this concept of attachment, and the need that individuals have for closeness while preserving a sense of self – Erikson's Intimacy versus Isolation, to which we referred at the beginning of the chapter – that we are now concerned.

In an excellent article, Morley (1982) takes Erikson's description as the starting point for what he sees as the central issues confronting couples in their relationships. Quoting *Marriage Matters* that 'at issue . . . [in marital problems is] what is conceived of as an actual or potential threat to the "self"' (Home Office 1979:22), he says:

> 'the necessity for an intimate other, or others, for psychological as well as physical health remains with us throughout life, and the struggle to be with as well as apart from that intimate relationship is perhaps part of the essence of being and in my view is certainly a fundamental aspect of the marital relationship and other intimate relationships which resemble marriage.'   (Morley 1982:13)

Thus although marriage is seen and experienced by many as potentially developmental, it also involves, for many people, a threat to self and an inhibition to self-development. There is often 'a fine balance of gains and losses to be negotiated' (Morley 1982:13).

Similarly, Askham argues that the marital relationship is one 'embodying a contradiction between identity and stability pursuit' (1984:194). She sees marriage as an identity-creating and therefore changing relationship, which also has to cope with the conflicting need for stability; these two contradictory functions produce potentially conflicting behaviours, which must be negotiated within the relationship. Jung (1925), in an interesting article, also views marriage as a kind of emotional container and emphasizes the task of individuation as a necessary if problematic stage in the working out of a marital relationship. There is further empirical support for this in a study of the patterns and processes of early marriage, which argues that

'the fact that first marriage was for many couples the official end of adolescence was striking. It is an interesting paradox that for these men and women part of the motive for matrimony is to experience independence and freedom. However, in order to achieve that independence they have become involved in a relationship which requires some level of dependence.'   (Mansfield 1982:11)

Morley (1982) sees the negotiations of gains and losses as taking place around factors that, extrapolated from Erikson's (1965) description, can be expressed in terms of pairs of opposing characteristics. Each need, felt and expressed, may also involve some threat of loss of self. Erikson's Intimacy versus Isolation he sees as covering four distinct issues, which need to be separated in order to be understood.

The first, *Attachment versus Detachment*, reflects Bowlby's formulations, but Morley draws attention to the way that attachment behaviour and the 'ebb and flow of anxiety' (1982:14) around the need to be attached go on throughout life. Clearly the extent to which early parental attachments were reliable and anxiety-free will influence the adult's ability to form secure attachments, but for all except the most damaged, who may be unable to form attachments at all, the attempt to find the position on the continuum of attachment–detachment that is most comfortable for them is a continuing one. As in the attachment behaviour of the child, the adult may exhibit it most powerfully when the external world becomes most threatening.

Morley describes the second element as *Commitment versus Disengagement*, referring thereby to the extension of relationships in time, 'as well as to concepts of exclusivity and promiscuity' (1982:15). He considers that many individuals experience the marriage contract, or the continuing of the marriage bond, as a threat to their ontological security, the struggle with the need to be committed and the anxiety that this creates in terms of their continued survival as separate people. The not uncommon problem, where couples who have been cohabiting successfully experience a distressing deterioration in their relationship when they marry, he attributes to anxiety about the loss of individual autonomy in a committed relationship. This was a problem that interested Dicks (1967), who explained it in terms of divergence from conformity to parental models of marriage. This is consistent with the notion of threat to self, since the self-structure is so closely bound up with identification with and sense of separateness from parental models. Some couples organize their lives in such a way as to preserve both commitment and disengagement in a relatively stable way – e.g. employment involving long absences away from home. Others, with less stability, break up and come together repeatedly.

The third element Morley discusses is the conflict between *Intimacy and Alienation*, which he considers the factor most powerful in its impact upon the self and its survival.

'The concept of self suggests a deep sense of inviolability and kind of inner core of privacy which is safe from intrusion and whose continued existence is secure. The notion of intimacy runs quite contrary to this and suggests a voluntary surrendering of privacy in favour of a profound sense of closeness with another.'   (Morley 1982:17)

Such closeness can be satisfying, with the feeling of being totally known and understood, but the exposure and acknowledgement of vulnerability can also be

'profoundly frightening to those whose sense of identity and selfhood is less securely held . . . . The penetrating proximity of the other threatens to dissolve the uncertain and insecure boundaries of the partners.'   (Morley 1982:18)

For some people, the desire for intimacy arouses such anxiety that it may be possible for them to attain it only within the context of a brief relationship. This, amongst other factors, may be at work in the repetitive patterns of brief relationships with 'unsuitable' or 'unavailable' partners.

The fourth element Morley identifies is *Similarity versus Difference*. Basing this on observation of the difficulties experienced in inter-racial marriages that were largely concerned with difference, he concluded that while such evident dissimilarity blocked off the possibility of closeness at one level, at another strangeness was erotic and sexually exciting. He hypothesizes that for those whose own sense of identity is poorly developed, the perceived differences may bring a sense of safety, in that the boundary of self would be maintained by the choice of a partner with whom it is impossible to identify closely. The issue of similarity and difference is not of course confined to this, and inter-racial marriages may be only at one end of the spectrum. Anxieties about gender difference are also encompassed by this dimension, in that at some level people have to deal with anxieties about sexual difference. Although, for perhaps most of us, the anxieties can be overcome, and successful heterosexual relationships formed, some cannot contemplate a sexual relationship with the opposite sex, whilst others 'assuage the anxiety aroused by the perception of genital difference by choosing partners sometimes of the same sex and sometimes not' (Morley 1982:19).

These different elements, all of which involve a conflict within themselves, may also be in conflict with each other. Thus for example, 'anxieties about commitment and their resolution by an approach towards disengagement may arouse fears about a loss of attachment' (Morley 1982:20), and so on.

It is evident that Morley is talking about aspects of the marital relationship to which we have already referred. This particular framework is useful since it draws attention to the self and the different avenues it takes for its survival. Furthermore, it illuminates many of the difficulties that we know clients experience. Where a worker is concerned, for example, to help and understand a client who is hesitantly moving towards establishing a relationship or is constantly moving from one relationship to another, it may be useful to think about this in terms of the issues it raises for the self regarding attachment, intimacy, and so on. Morley's formulations draw attention to the non-pathological concerns that affect all couples and emphasize attachment behaviour, which we consider crucial in understanding marital relationships. They also lead to a consideration of the myriad dimensions of daily life in which these concerns are enacted and worked out. Furthermore, the opposing characteristics remind us of the dynamic rather than the static nature of the self and the relationships between the self and others. The potential usefulness of these concepts for social-work practice will be explored in the final section of this chapter.

Finally, a number of psychodynamically based attempts to classify marital problems have been made, which may be found helpful in organizing ideas about the nature of these difficulties. These are

reviewed by Berman and Lief (1975) in a useful article in which they
identify four main types of classificatory system: the first being based
on rules of power, the second on parental stage and the presence or
absence of children, and the third and fourth on the level of intimacy
and complementary fit.

Systems approaches

Gorrell Barnes, in her book about working with families, describes the
way in which 'the patterning of daily life in any family is built up over
the lifetime of the current family and incorporates what has been
learnt from the patterns of previous generations' (1984a:5).

The idea of the family as a system is based on this view of it as an organization that over time has developed its own patterns, habits, and rules
of behaviour. Therapists working from a systems perspective have
founded their ideas about marital interaction and intervention on this
view. In order to make sense of what appeared to be patterns of behaviour that recurred, despite variations in detail, in the interactions of
different families, concepts based on general systems theory have been
utilized as a means of organizing these observations. Since systems
theory represents the most coherent conceptualization of these processes of interaction, some discussion of the main propositions and their
application to marital interaction is appropriate.

Three points should be made concerning this discussion. First,
although the theorists who are commonly identified with this
perspective base some of their ideas on a general systems approach
and make some similar basic assumptions, they focus on different
aspects of family interaction. Thus, although the major systems
approaches – the strategic therapy of Jay Haley, the Palo Alto model,
Minuchin's structural family therapy, the theories of Bowen, the
eclectic communications therapy of Satir, and the Milan model –
have ideas in common, their analysis and practice are often divergent.
This need not concern practitioners unduly, except in so far as it
makes their ideas harder to synthesize and to utilize.

A second dilemma in discussing this orientation in a book on
marital work is in deciding the extent to which the concepts of all the
principal systems theorists should be reviewed. Their ideas have had a
major impact on family work in Britain; and in so far as the couple is
seen as part of the family, systems concepts must necessarily influence
thinking about couple relationships as well. On the other hand, in a
systems approach, the marital dyad is seen as a sub-system of the

family, and with certain exceptions the majority of theorists have focussed on the two- (or three-) generational family system, rather than on the marital system itself. Further consideration of the issue of working with the couple in the context of the family is given in Chapter 4; the present discussion will therefore concentrate on those writers who have concerned themselves specifically with working with the marital dyad. A further reason for this is that systems approaches to family work have gained wide acceptance in Britain, and there are a number of accounts of it readily available (e.g. Gorrell Barnes 1984b).

Thirdly, there is some terminological confusion in the use of the terms 'general systems theory' and 'family systems theories'. It would be inaccurate and misleading, as Gurman (1978) points out, to assert that 'systems' therapies are based entirely or even substantially on general systems theories, for there are numerous family systems theories varying in the degree to which they adhere or deviate from general systems theory. Equally, marital therapy was established as a systems-orientated approach long before it adopted some of the family systems themes.

General systems theory has however been the source of some important ideas for family systems theory. It contends that there are certain fundamental characteristics of organizational systems that are common to all systems and can be delineated and generalized across systems, irrespective of content. A major distinction in general systems theory is whether one is dealing with an open system, where exchanges are allowed across boundaries, or a closed system, where they are not. Since all living systems are open systems, it follows that,

'in contrast to equilibrium states in closed systems which are determined by initial conditions, the open system may attain a time-independent state, independent of initial conditions and determined only by the system parameters.'   (Von Bertalanffy 1962:7)

As Segraves (1982) shows, this concept, which is central to the work of the major systems theorists, involves an important perceptual shift from the psychoanalytic approach, which regards marriage as a closed system, with the relationship determined by the initial personalities of the partners. Subsequent systems theorists have refined the concept of openness, to make it more useful in describing the complexity of family systems. Thus:

'one can imagine a continuum moving from the relatively open . . . to the relatively closed family system, engaged in minimal

interchange with either its suprasystem or its sub-systems.'
                                        (Walrond-Skinner 1976:13)

A system is described as a complex set of elements existing in some consistent relationship with each other. To understand an interactional system, one has to determine the interrelationship of these elements, so that the system cannot be understood once it has been broken down into its separate parts. Hence the system concept of *wholeness*; i.e. a system has a life and a force of its own that are more than the sum of its parts. Similarly, a change in one part of the system invariably leads to a change elsewhere in it. A second generating concept of systems theory is that of *circular causality*. In a close interpersonal relationship such as marriage, each partner's behaviour is viewed as a reaction or adjustment to the behaviour of the other. One partner nags because the second is distant and withdrawn, and the other withdraws because the first nags. From this perspective, the behaviour occurring between the couple is produced and maintained by both. Since the causal circle is one in which all elements of the behaviour occur in the present, the past and intra-psychic factors assume less centrality.

Any system of components existing in a consistent relationship must be marked by a boundary, which circumscribes its identity and distinguishes it from other systems and its external environment. Skynner (1976), in discussing this systems concept, highlights the importance of understanding the system's boundaries and their crucial function both in restricting and in allowing exchange across them. Central also to Minuchin's (1974) thinking on marriage is that, in order to survive and develop, the marital sub-system must have clearly defined boundaries to protect it from intrusion from competing sub-systems, such as children or families of origin.

There are a number of other systems concepts that have influenced family and marital therapists. The term 'negentropy' refers to the way in which energy can be brought in and out of a system, leading to growth and development and an increased degree of organization and lessening of disarray. By analogy, this concept has led theorists to be concerned with the interactions between family systems and the environment, and the flow of information and communication between the marital and family systems. 'Isomorphism' refers 'to the presence of similar structures in seemingly dissimilar systems' (Segraves 1982:81); in marital therapy it is used to describe the apparently oppositional behaviour of the couple, which none the less serves the function of maintaining the system at the same point.

'Homeostasis', a term referred to in Chapter 2, is commonly used to describe those feedback schemes that serve to maintain the system as it is. Systems theorists have used the concept as a way of describing and understanding the repetitive nature of many patterns of interaction within families. For example, Watzlawick, Beavin, and Jackson (1967) discuss a couple who, despite frequent arguments about each other's remoteness, seemed to maintain a constant level of intimacy in their behaviour. When one tried to reach out, the other would withdraw, and at other times the roles would be reversed. They argue that the homeostasis of the system was maintained by a hypothetical feedback loop, which served to keep the intimacy at a more or less constant level. In other words, the system resists individuals' efforts to change and prescribes the members' behaviours to adapt to the needs of the system.

In positive feedback the error is self-enhancing, whereas in negative feedback error is utilized to correct error. Thus Rapoport writes that with positive feedback 'either a variable increases without bound or vacillations of ever increasing amplitude result' (1974:1088). Lederer and Jackson (1968) and Watzalwick, Beavin, and Jackson (1967) use this concept to describe the kind of escalating struggles that occur between couples, where each increment in anger further increases the struggle, Lederer and Jackson describing this situation as a 'runaway', and Watzlawick as a 'game without end'.

Closely connected to the concept of homeostasis is the view of the system or sub-system of the family as governed either explicitly or implicitly by family rules or norms. These may best be understood perhaps by the idea of habits or customs, which families inevitably develop as an economical means of handling the myriad interactions that occur in daily life. These function to enable members of the system to interact economically without needing to return constantly to first principles of behaviour, and to anticipate and predict reactions of other members of the system. At a simple and obvious level such rules might, for example, enable a family to sit down and eat together without having to decide on each occasion the timing of the meal, acceptable behaviour, who cooks, who clears away, and so on. At a subtler level, families develop customs or rules about such things as the expression of anger, appreciation, or affection, how decisions are made within the family, and the part each member takes in the interaction, all of which are essential parts of assessing marital interaction from a systems point of view. The Milan School in particular emphasizes the importance of understanding the rules and norms governing the family's behaviour, and of the interlinking of the events themselves and the perceptions and meanings given to

those events by the family members. In contrast to the change orientation of most approaches, here the therapists work from a strictly
neutral stance of observation, playing back to the family what they
have understood of its functioning but with no explicit requirement
for change (Palazolli *et al.* 1978).

As we suggest above, systems theorists have focussed on the marital
relationship to varying degrees. In Minuchin's (1974) structural model,
for example, marriage is analysed in terms of three dimensions of its
structure: its organizational characteristics (membership and boundaries), the pattern of its transitions over time, and its response to stress.
Although discussing the marital dyad in some detail, Minuchin concentrates on the two-generational system, whilst we are more concerned
here with the dyad. Jackson, Haley, and Satir, however, whose work is
associated to various degrees with the Palo Alto Mental Health Institute, have each been particularly influential in the field of marital therapy with couples, and their contributions are therefore worth reviewing.

Jackson's (1977) orientation to marriage and marital work is an interactional one, and reflects the pioneer work that he carried out in the
study of communication patterns in the families of schizophrenics. His
approach may be best understood in two of his key concepts, that of the
marital quid pro quo, and that of *communication*. The notion of rules
explicitly or implictly governing the behaviour of individuals within a
family system has already been referred to. Jackson postulates that, in
the early stages of a couple relationship, a kind of bargaining process
takes place in which each spouse attempts to define and establish the
relationship to their advantage. Assuming that the relationship continues, this struggle to reach a mutually agreed position about each
spouse's relationship to the other stabilizes:

> 'these relationship agreements ... prescribe and limit the individ-
> ual's behaviour over a wide variety of content areas, organising
> their interaction into a reasonably stable system.'
>
> (Jackson 1977:9)

Thus the partners will develop a series of implicit rules by which they
determine, among other things, who is to have control in which situations and what each is to give or allow in return for what. However, this
metaphorical 'bargain', which Jackson refers to as the marital quid pro
quo, denotes more than just negotiations over specific content issues,
since it involves some notion of self-definition, leading to a requirement
about the behaviour of the other. This is in some ways similar to the idea
of 'fit' postulated by the object relations theorists.

Haley (1963), developing this idea of negotiating rules in the early stages of marriage, considers that conflict over these can occur at three levels: the rules themselves, who has the right to set the rules, and enforcement of incompatible rules or ambiguous communication about rules. Since individuals' expectations of marriage often derive from the implicit rules in their families of origin, conflict will often arise from the struggle to reconcile these differing assumptions, a process that may be painful but is often in fact soluble. These struggles, about 'who is to tell whom what to do under what circumstances' (Haley 1963:227), are the source of major conflicts in marriage, and Haley describes in detail the nuances and tactics of such struggles.

With both Jackson and Haley, a central theme is the effort of partners to control the relationship and to circumscribe the range of each other's behaviour. They argue that therapy should therefore aim to change the rules of behaviour and focus on interventions at a transactional rather than individual level, which are designed to interrupt recurring sequences of behaviour. A principal task must also consist of examining and modifying the communication patterns by which rules of behaviour are established and maintained. Jackson draws attention to the complexity of communication between partners, and the possibility of misunderstanding occurring at the levels at which it operates, since 'communication always necessarily involves a multiplicity of messages of different levels, at once' (Jackson and Weakland 1971:16). For example, communication can be conceptualized as consisting of both a content level and a relationship level, and many disagreements between couples apparently about content may in fact be about relationship difficulties that are never explicitly acknowledged. One manifestation of this with which readers will be familiar, through the writings of R.D. Laing, is the concept of the double bind, where the content communication contradicts the communication at the meta- or relationship level.

Satir's (1967) main contribution in the field of marital therapy has lain in emphasizing the importance of clear communication in resolving interpersonal difficulties. She postulates that people need to have a secure and distinct sense of self and other. Failure to achieve this is partly attributable to a failure to identify and distinguish between internal feelings and external reality, the tendency to confuse these, to project feelings, and not to discriminate between objective fact and personal belief about that fact. These confusions about assumptive worlds, states, and perceptions are a major source of difficulty between people; and a partial solution to such difficulties is for people 'to learn and employ clear language that differentiates self from other and to use explicit language that limits the amount of distortion and projection possible' (Segraves 1978:451−552). Good communication requires a differentiation between self and other, with clarity and congruence between levels of communication. Common communication problems, which are seen as violating these principles, include 'mind-reading', incomplete messages, generalizing, vague referents and indirect anger, cross-complaining, and channel inconsistency. Helping couples disentangle these is a major thrust in the intervention offered by both systems theorists and behaviourists, and the approach will be explored in detail in Chapter 5.

There are certain problems with the contributions of systems theorists to the field. First, some of the assumptions of writers such as Jackson and Haley in particular, and the language in which they are couched − e.g. the jokey labels such as 'gruesome twosome', 'weary wranglers' − seem distasteful. The central theme of the Jackson and Haley approach, which emphasizes the efforts of partners to control the relationship and the gambits, games, subterfuges, deceptions, and ploys that they use in order to do so, appears to embody a derogatory and diminishing view of individuals and their interactions, which social workers may find unpalatable.

Secondly, the view of the complexity with which messages are delivered, and the notion of good communication as being exemplified by statements such as 'I want this from you in this situation' (Satir 1967:87), denies such values as altruism, unselfishness, and self-denial a legitimate place in the individual's repertoire. Since many of the human potential books on the market − from *I'm OK, You're OK* (Harris 1973) onward − with their injunctions to 'live in your own space', 'take responsibility for your own actions', etc., are offshoots of this thinking, its influence is widespread and by no means entirely helpful. An interesting alternative perspective to this is offered by Askham (1984), who found that couples often withheld comments and utterances in the interests of preserving the relationship.

Thirdly, it seems to us possible to couch the major contributions and assumptions of these theorists in language that would convey the same meaning but avoid the distancing and mystifying effect of much systems terminology. For example, as far back as 1955 Kelly in his work on personal constructs argued that behaviour and the inner representational model, set, or 'construct' were reciprocally related to each other, so that change in the former might produce change in the interpersonal world and vice versa. Similarly, other cognitive social psychologists have drawn attention to the circular way in which certain kinds of behaviour produce certain kinds of response, and to the fact that these may be self-perpetuating. We would agree with Segraves (1982) that the four major propositions of the systems theorists could be summarized as follows, thus avoiding the alien and perhaps pseudo-scientific language of systems terminology:

- that current interpersonal transactions are prime determinants of the personality of the individual;
- that the exchanges between a couple are circular rather than having a linear causality;
- that many of these exchanges are self-perpetuating and difficult for the couple themselves to check; and
- that behaviour change (in which we include change in patterns or style of communication) may be therapeutic, and affect the world of those involved.

Behavioural approaches

Behavioural approaches to marital difficulties are based on social learning principles and tend to view the marital relationship in terms of the mutual behaviour shaping it. As with systems theories, they emphasize the current situational determinants of behaviour, and assume that interpersonal difficulties may be understood by identifying those factors in the present situation that perpetuate these difficulties. Since these may be ameliorated by changing these factors, the focus is on current as opposed to past behaviour. An important contribution of the behavioural marital therapists has been their commitment to demonstrating their propositions empirically. We do not propose to review the basic concepts of behavioural or social learning approaches to human problems, and some familiarity with these is assumed. Weiss (1978) offers a useful and comprehensive review of the basic principles and techniques of behaviour modification before discussing their application to marital difficulties, to which the reader is referred.

The impact of the social exchange theorists, such as Thibaut and Kelley (1959) and Homans (1961), is evident in the work of most behavioural marital therapists. Social exchange theorists apply a kind of behavioural economics to the field of human relationships, and assume that every interpersonal transaction can be understood in terms of the costs and benefits to the participants. In any dyadic relationship, according to Thibaut and Kelley, participants attempt to maximize the rewards of the exchange while minimizing the costs.

Thus to be successful, a relationship must have a higher reward/cost ratio than other competing relationships or activities available to the individuals at the time. A form of reciprocity develops over time, so that, when rewards and costs become unbalanced, the participants attempt to restore equilibrium.

The exchange model is slightly more complex when applied to couples. In a satisfying marriage,

> 'not only should the intrinsically beneficial behaviours be low cost to the other, but each person must receive high beneficial behaviours from the other; it follows that one person's received beneficial behaviours should also be low cost (therefore easier to give) behaviours to the other!'   (Thibaut and Kelley 1959:49)

In other words, if the washing-up is done extremely unwillingly, only because the other person wants it, very negative feelings are going to result. The fact that this kind of exchange is so interdependent means that each person must have a potentially high regard for the other. In a successful marriage, therefore, the rewards that are worked for are mutual ones, while the costs that are minimized are individual. Askham's (1984) view of marriage as a balance between the costs in terms of the sacrifice of identity development and the rewards to do with the achievement of stability seems to reflect a similar dynamic.

There is also some empirical support for the notion that in unhappy marriages the costs are high relative to the rewards. Birchler (1973) found that couples in distressed marriages reported fewer exchanges of rewarding behaviour (quoted in Segraves 1982:108). Similarly, lower rates of what are presumably rewarding behaviours, such as recreational activities, talking, and sex, have also been found (Stuart 1969, Weiss, Birchler, and Vincent 1974), although these studies have been criticized on methodological grounds.

A concept related to this is that in unhappy marriages, because the costs are higher than the rewards, the exchange process changes to one where the emphasis is on minimizing individual costs with little apparent expectation of reward. A coercive control system develops, in which one person tries to coerce positive behaviour in exchange for negative reinforcements. Coercion is considered to be a high-cost behaviour since it usually produces reciprocal aversive behaviour in response, and is thus self-defeating. For example, a wife seeking greater expression of love and affection from her husband may become angry and abusive when this is not forthcoming, making him even less likely to respond to her with affection.

Although working with slightly differing formulations of the genesis and maintenance of marital problems, most behavioural therapists approach marital discord from some principles of operant conditioning. Thus, the fact that most distressed couples use negative reinforcement as a means of trying to change behaviour is seen as a key factor. Following operant conditioning principles, positive reinforcement is held to be a more effective change mechanism, so this is seen as a crucial error in most disturbed marriages. However, the fact that each partner partially controls the behaviour of the other by the contingencies he or she establishes for the behaviour, so that therapeutic change requires a simultaneous change in both spouses, is a complication in the application of the operant conditioning approach to working with unhappy marriages.

In addition to faulty reinforcement behaviour, marriages may become distressed because of what is called a communication deficit – i.e. when a communication is received in a way that was not intended. The deficit exists, as Weiss (1978) points out, only when intention and impact do not agree, not when they are both negative. 'A wife intending to send negative and husband receiving negative have a problem with negatives, not with communications' (Weiss 1978:188).

Finally, many of the formulations of behavioural principles relating to marriage mention cognitive variables, at least to the extent that they are beginning to incorporate ideas about the role of expectations and the building of sentiments. For example, Jacobson and Margolin stress cognitive evaluation as part of their initial assessment of the couple:

'Spouses enter therapy with numerous assumptions about what has caused their marital problems, with evaluations of their mates as marital partners and with attitudes about the quality of the relationship. These cognitions play an important role.' (1979:70–1)

The goal of behavioural work with marital problems is to provide couples with behaviour-change operations based on positive control procedures, two principal approaches to which may be distinguished. The first involves teaching positive reinforcement procedures – in other words, helping couples bargain more effectively with each other through contracting, reciprocity counselling, and negotiation training, for example. The second involves improving faulty communication patterns through the teaching of communication skills. A detailed account of these approaches follows in Chapter 5.

The application of behavioural approaches to marriage and

marital therapy is not without problems. The approach is essentially, although not entirely, ahistorical and takes the view that marital behaviour is based largely on the immediate present behaviour of the other spouse. This view takes little account of the common observation of those working in the field that many people repeat, in subsequent intimate relationships, problem behaviours experienced in earlier such relationships. This points to the existence of at least some individual characterological difficulties within intimate relationships.

There is also the assumption that marital difficulties arise from faulty behaviour-change mechanisms, and that conflict occurs because the demand behaviour from one partner is met with non-compliance in some way by the other. Unsuccessful marriages are therefore characterized by a lack of reciprocity between the couple. Detailed criticisms of the concept of reciprocity have been made, however (Gottman *et al.* 1976, Segraves 1982), and this view of marital difficulties again seems to contradict much everyday experience. For example, in Iris Murdoch's *The Sacred and Profane Love Machine* (1974), there are no overt problems between the married couple, and Harriet, the wife, makes no demand for immediate change in the behaviour of her husband; but the satisfaction that he derives in his well-disguised extramarital relationship through the passive – aggressive expression of hostility is evident, and ultimately the marriage breaks down.

In addition, there are difficulties with the view that change in the behaviour of one will produce corresponding changes in the way he or she is perceived by the other. 'When one changes his behaviour, there are corresponding changes in the other's impressions and perceptions of him' (Stuart 1969:677). This, as Gurman points out, is 'simply incomplete, even from a social learning point of view' (1978:486). An 'impression' is based on the other's behaviour as interpreted through the individual's perceptual system. A change in one person's behaviour may alter the other's perceptions, but since these problem behaviours will probably occur in areas of real difficulty and sensitivity, the chances are that changes in them will not in fact alter the other's perception of them. Given the nature of intimate relationships, and the way in which they involve deep-set anxieties and conflicts, modifying interpersonal attitudes is more problematic than the emphasis on the techniques of behaviour change might suggest.

There may be unexpected spin-offs from this focussing on concrete issues. A couple who were locked in a bitter struggle over the perceived failures of each to do what the other considered desirable moved quite rapidly, after an attempt to modify the behaviours, to recognizing that these behaviours were not in fact the issue at all. For others, the behavioural exchange model with its emphasis on the responsibility for the self, and bartering between separate psychological entities, may in fact be helpful in enabling an enmeshed couple to establish a clearer sense of self, and more realistic expectations of marriage. Segraves also points out that

'Many psychodynamic therapists have as a goal the establishment of clear "ego boundaries" or the interpretation and resolution of projection systems in disturbed marriages. The behavioural exchange model could be construed as a concretisation of this goal.'
(1982:119)

The other difficulty in accepting this model in its entirety is that is seems to reflect a view of couples in conflict as rational beings, committed to their relationship, who recognize the part that each plays in producing the marital conflict. Where in all this is the much more familiar appli- cant to the social-work agency? Alone and female, she presents herself as vaguely depressed or sometimes more seriously ill, and her partner, when he comes, is there only to help the identified patient. And where is the partner who regales the worker with a list of the faults and fail- ings of the spouse, with little or no perception that he might have some responsibility for what has happened in the marriage? Behav- ioural exchanges would seem to involve both a commitment to the re- lationship over and above the needs of the two individuals, an accept- ance of a 'give-to-get' philosophy, and a recognition of mutual res- ponsibility in conflict. Merely the acceptance of such a philosophy would seem frequently sufficient in itself to produce an amelioration of the marital difficulties.

Summary

The final section of this chapter will attempt to extract from these dif- ferent approaches some organizing principles and concepts to help people working with distressed couples. As we argued earlier, we assume a fairly general readiness amongst British social workers to accept this approach, and a distaste for the generally sterile argu- ments over rival theoretical approaches that are more characteristic of American debate. We have taken as the basis of our selection Lewis's oft-quoted aphorism that 'there is nothing so practical as a good theory', and have tried to select those ideas that seem best to explain or at least address common problems faced by the practitioner. Our selection must to some extent be personal, but there seems to be a mechanism that operates with theory in social work, whereby some concepts are found to be useful and pass into common parlance, whilst others that do not are discarded – the different fate of the now colloquial 'defence mechanism' and the neglected 'Oedipus complex', both originating from Freud, are a case in point.

First, it is valuable to have some notion of what are common issues for couples. A useful starting point for this is to think of a couple or pair as two people, whose behaviour is explicable to some degree by that of their partner. Common couple concerns are those arising from this interrelatedness, and are to do with the way in which the self retains its own sense of individuality, selfdom, and integrity, while fulfilling a basic psychological and biological need to be attached to another. Morley's (1982) delineation of four different facets of this and the attempt to balance needs that are in some sense in opposition seems most helpful in this context. Thus, in the not uncommon situation where one partner takes on the role of pursuer while the other withdraws, it is helpful to think of them as having essentially split responsibility for two 'classic couple issues' (Wile 1981). One has taken on the part of attempting to maintain intimacy and commitment and detecting its absence, while the other takes responsibility for voicing their mutual need to preserve their separate individuality by maintaining a measure of detachment and difference.

This development of ideas around Erikson's notion of Intimacy versus Isolation has particular relevance to those situations where the problem is not so much the maintenance of an existing relationship, but one of a pattern of serial relationships with intimate others. It also has the merit of offering a radical and non-judgemental means of understanding the different ways of relating to each other and styles of living through which couples, faced with a lack of constraints from society, work out the problems of this relationship. Minuchin's emphasis on understanding the way in which the couple is responding to stress, and his view that stress is an inevitable part of the life of a couple, is also a useful one. Equally, his use of the systems concept of boundaries offers a slightly different but illuminating perspective on an aspect of this classic couple issue of being part of, but also separate from, other family and social systems.

Secondly, it is evident that concepts are required that allow some understanding of the interplay between the current circumstances and transactions of the relationship, and the individual characters and histories of the partners, whether or not this understanding is used directly in work with them. For example, using the illustration of the couple dynamic mentioned above, which partner becomes the seeker and which the withdrawer is partly determined by their individual histories. A husband's sensitivity to his wife's pursuit may be partly based on early experiences of an over-protecting and engulfing mother, while her sensitivity to her husband's withdrawing may be built on experiences of rejection by one of her intimate carers when she was young. Such awareness may not necessarily be used in direct discussion with the couple, but a conceptual framework that allows one to understand how such factors influence the management of closeness and distance in the present relationship is necessary. The contributions to the understanding of marital discord of the psychodynamically orientated therapists are of major importance here, since the ideas of projective identification, transference, and collusion address themselves to the problem of how individuals' past experiences become internalized and then continue to be worked out in current intimate relationships. They also offer explanations about how people can behave so differently in intimate adult relationships from other adult relationships, since they are concerned with the re-creation of the past in the present. Allied to this is the need to understand why individuals are drawn to particular partners in the first place. Dicks's ideas about the three levels on which this choice is made, and the development of these by other writers from the IMS, offer, in our view, the fullest account of this process, with the caveat that their subsequent work has tended to concentrate somewhat restrictively on unconscious choices.

Thirdly, it seems important to have some explanatory hypothesis about the phenomenon of the distorted perceptions that distressed couples often have of each other. The work of the object relations theorists can contribute to our understanding of how and why this occurs, and the behaviourists and systems theorists are a fruitful source of ideas concerning the part that communication and specific behaviours play in maintaining these misperceptions.

Fourthly, systems thinking emphasizes in an important way the manner in which habits, attitudes, perceptions, and customs develop in families and function as a kind of shorthand, enabling them to live together without returning to first principles over each issue. It also highlights the idea of the couple as a system or sub-system, so that the behaviour of each becomes to some extent explicable in terms of the other, and what is done to one member of the system affects the others. The concept of homeostasis draws attention to the tendency of systems to resist change, and has perhaps served to organize thinking around this area and encourage practitioners to work at particular ways of dealing with it – e.g. by the 'reframing' ideas discussed in Chapter 5.

It may be argued, however, that in the context of systems theory and family work there has been much ado about comparatively little. Systems terminology is not necessary to explain the ways in which couples and families resist change. The central idea of systems thinking, that the focus should or could be the relationship rather than the individual, is also implicit in object relations thinking. To call this, as Walrond-Skinner (1979) does, a 'unique' insight is to ignore the contributions of the other approaches.

Finally, the conceptual framework of the theory of personal constructs, drawn from cognitive social psychology, may provide a useful conceptual bridge between object relations theory on the one hand and systems and behaviour theory on the other – and, for social workers, a means of translating some esoteric ideas into prescriptions for action. The essence of this framework is the assumption that people develop a series of what may be called 'templates', or 'perceptual goggles', with which they sense and organize the present environment and current reality. These perceptions – or, as Kelly (1955) called them, 'constructs' – are determined by current reality and past experiences in similar situations, and are therefore internal representational schema of discrete portions of the universe, generated by individuals from their experience of it, which enable them to organize their experience and anticipate reality:

> '[They] can be considered as a kind of scanning pattern which a person continually projects upon his world. As he sweeps back and forth across his perceptual field he picks up blips of meaning. The more adequate his scanning pattern, the more meaningful his world becomes.'　　　　　　　　　　　　　　　　(Kelly 1955:145)

This concept of 'personal constructs' is useful, first, because it avoids becoming entangled in certain of the assumptions of the ideas about ego split and so on. Second, because it allows ideas about individual history, assumptive world, family habits and customs, and their conjunction with present experience to be combined in a way that a behavioural model does not. Third, because it allows for the modification of personal 'schema', perceptions, and assumptions by direct behavioural disconfirmation, which the psychodynamic model does not easily include. Fourth, because it allows that this may occur by verbal persuasion and by changing the manner in which people communicate. And fifth, because it addresses itself to the question, seen by many therapists to be a pivotal one, of the misperceptions of the spouse's character and motivations in the genesis and maintenance of marital discord. It thus becomes possible to assess the couple's mutual behaviour, either as (a) understandable reactions to present circumstances, thus freeing us from the tendency to emphasize the pathological, which is a feature of the object relations approach; or (b) particular difficulties around common couple concerns, as Morley (1982) delineates them; or (c) distorted expressions of the ordinary adult needs involved (Wile 1981).

We have argued in this final section that practitioners may be helped by having some idea of common couple issues, some means of conceptualizing the habitual distortions of perceptions and communication between couples, and some understanding of the interplay between the individual and his current family life and environment. We have also indicated points at which the contributions of objects relations theory, systems approaches, and behavioural approaches may be helpful in understanding marital problems, and we have suggested that the idea of personal constructs may be useful in making a bridge between past and internal psychological events, and current observable interpersonal ones. In Part II of the book we shall explore how the explanatory concepts offered and the understanding achieved so far can be translated into practice.

Note

1 We acknowledge this observation to Mrs E.E. Irvine.

Working with marital problems

4

Deciding to work with marital problems

The second part of this book concentrates on working with marital relationships, which necessitates facing up to the untidiness of real problems and the lack of adequate theoretical explanations which might lead to clear prescriptions for practice. From the outset, practical issues such as the difficulty of focussing on the marital dyad, or of deciding whether or not to maintain this focus or to work with the family, will need to be recognized and contended with. This is our purpose in this chapter.

Archer (1982) lucidly describes such problems in her detailed account of work with a married couple. The initial referral concerns a woman, without her husband, the client's initial acknowledgement of marital problems being minimal – the marriage is simply 'over' (1982:151). Early intervention involves the couple as separate individuals, and there is considerable investment in the worker–wife relationship. When work is undertaken with the couple, other work at the boundary (e.g. with the education welfare officer) continues; the children are included in one important session by chance, as indeed is the co-worker in an emergency night interview. In her discussion, Archer suggests that there remain questions about her analysis of the situation, and wonders, 'Would it have been preferable to have taken one clear theoretical perspective right from the beginning and followed that line, that one method of working?' (1982:165)

It was argued in Chapter 3, however, that none of the major theoretical perspectives is adequate on its own to explain problems in marital relationships. Consequently, as we shall suggest in Chapter 5, there is no single set of prescriptions for practice that can be derived from any one of these perspectives and then applied to marital problems. And yet

Archer's uncertainty, reflecting a lack of clarity and sense of direction in her attempts to help – with which all social workers will be familiar – represents one of the major problems confronting social work.

This particular difficulty stems primarily from the range and complexity of the influences contributing to marital problems, which were discussed in Part I. The analysis of marital problems therefore requires an approach that takes account of the complexity of such a reality and recognizes marital relationships as dynamic systems (or sub-systems of family systems) which influence and are influenced by a variety of both internal and external pressures. Perhaps the best-known application of general systems theory, which was discussed in Chapter 3, to social work is that offered by Pincus and Minahan (1973). This approach, which may not only help to clarify the most complex of problems, but also suggest various possibilities for intervention, is designed 'to provide a common base of knowledge, values and skills for professional social workers in any organisation that delivers services to people or in any field of practice' (Pincus and Minahan 1977:74). Such an approach is particularly suited to our purpose and we shall refer to it in subsequent sections.

The model is built around the interaction of four systems (for a fuller discussion of these, the reader is referred to Pincus and Minahan 1973 and 1977):

1 the change-agent system – the social worker and the agency to which they belong;
2 the client system – the person or family that engages the services of the worker and is expected to benefit from the worker's efforts;
3 the target system – those people the social worker aims to influence in order to achieve the goals of intervention; and
4 the action system – the social worker and the people worked with in order to achieve the goals of intervention.

In much of the discussion that follows, we will be concerned primarily with the target system and the action system, particularly the latter, decisions about which often present a major dilemma for the social worker. An awareness of the other systems is important, however, since their interaction is central to the model and highlights the importance of understanding issues concerning worker, organization, and client – which, although we consider them separately, are in reality closely interwoven.

The anxieties of the social worker

The particular anxieties that practitioners may experience in working with marital problems have been widely acknowledged. We have already discussed the way in which the specialist literature on marital work may exacerbate social workers' doubts about their competence in this field. Brannen and Collard's (1982) findings about the difficulties clients have in disclosing aspects of their marital relationship suggest that the recipient of such disclosures may experience similar feelings of embarrassment and constraint. As *Marriage Matters* points out:

> 'marital work is particularly anxiety-provoking since the subject of marital relationships and sexual problems can touch off deep resonances in the worker relating to his own family experience.'
> (Home Office 1979:141)

We discussed in Chapter 3 the way the marital relationship touches upon core issues to do with the integrity of self; important though such things as parenting, or looking after elderly or handicapped relatives, may be in triggering anxieties about identification in individual workers, the process of distancing oneself from them and distinguishing their impact on the worker is easier than with marital problems. As in any helping relationship, the resonances that are touched will vary greatly between workers, but the fact that the marital relationship is an adult one based on choice also presupposes continuing transactions around that choice, which make it more likely to be an area of current sensitivity. It is also possible, given the increasing incidence of divorce, that a social worker may have to guard against the transference of feelings relating to the breakdown of their parents' or other close relatives' marriage. As Murch has indicated,

> 'The breakdown and stress in other people's family relationships can easily, through a process of projective identification, activate the practitioner's own inner fantasy world and arouse stress and anxiety.'   (1980:244)

Even general feelings of uncertainty and lack of confidence can be projected and inhibit a client from disclosing a problem. The positive side of this resonance is that, provided the worker recognizes any tendency to identify with the client's feelings and is careful to register and reflect upon personal reactions and feelings aroused, they may bring an immediacy of understanding to the problem that may be lacking in work with other difficulties.

Organizational issues

The worker's own hesitation about focussing on marital problems may be compounded by a lack of support from the agency. The process of shifting the focus to 'allow and encourage the marital partner to explore and express their difficulty' (Tebboth 1981:13) may involve subtle shifts of role for a worker in a non-specialist agency and the abandoning of the authority that provided the original basis for intervention. As Kahn and Earle have indicated, the difficulty of these early stages is that 'when the worker has no other assignment than to offer care and support . . . [this] is the precise moment when he himself is in most need of that care and support' (1982:126). If the agency is not organized in such a way as to provide this, or if the attitude towards such work is ambivalent, or if team seniors are themselves lacking in knowledge and expertise, the worker is unlikely to receive the kind of support and encouragement needed to move into difficult areas, for which there is no statutory authority, and about which both worker and clients may feel uncertain.

The significance of organizational factors in determining whether or not a marital problem is identified and actually worked with has been discussed in Chapter 2. Intake procedures, the orientation of social services departments towards cases where there are clear duties or services needed, and the difficulty experienced by workers in organizing their time in order to enable them to carry out sustained and regular work, all militate against a focus on complex emotional issues such as marital problems. Mattinson and Sinclair (1979) also point to the tendency of legal and bureaucratic frameworks to encourage the apportioning of blame in dealing with families under stress; this makes it harder for the worker to retain a focus on the marital interaction rather than on the individuals and to struggle against the natural human tendency to deal with stressful situations by apportioning blame:

> 'The law the social workers are administering is essentially concerned with need, as with the disabled, or blame, as with delinquency, or madness, which hovers uneasily between blame and need. . . . In practice, the designation of an individual as needy or blame-worthy often points the finger at a second individual.'
>
> (Mattinson and Sinclair 1979:283–84)

The operation of these regulations also contributed to what Mattinson and Sinclair describe as the 'segmental structure' of many of the married cases, which meant that social workers rarely saw husbands and wives together and that 'they would be particularly unlikely to do so where there were marital problems' (1979:309).

Similarly, in spite of the traditional involvement of the probation service in marital work, increasing emphasis is being placed on the provision of community alternatives to custody and on an increasingly explicit offence focus in social enquiry work. This, together with increased questioning of traditional casework methods with the consequent growth of pragmatic approaches to problem-solving, and the sharp decline in identifiable marital referrals, all add organizational pressures to the factors already referred to in Chapter 2, which result in probation officers being less likely to respond to marital problems than they might have been in the past.

When working in an agency that is not organized to support such activity, the worker may need to make the organization itself the target for change, as suggested in *Figure 1*.

Client perspective

If an agency emphasizes the provision of a particular kind of service, then clients are likely to respond to this. The uncertainties and ambiguities involved for clients in seeking and receiving help from social-work agencies have already been highlighted, and clients have some expectations of the kind of service or contact that will be provided, and may modify their requests or disclosures accordingly. Mattinson and Sinclair (1979) point to the difficulty, with clients whose experience of social service departments has been of work directed towards material and practical issues, of shifting the focus of work to one concerned with emotional issues. Brannen and Collard (1982) suggest that the client's uncertainties about acknowledging emotional problems may stem in part from previous situations involving disclosure of intensely personal and emotional problems, where a helper may have been found less than helpful. Clients who identify the agency with the exercise of statutory authority may be reluctant to admit to problems that might lead a social worker to doubt their competence. Indeed, even in an agency such as a Family Service Unit, where the workers are well known and there are certain guarantees about explicitness and openness, clients may increasingly see them as agents of social control concerned with child neglect and abuse, rather than as benevolent counsellors.

To this wariness about the potential power of social workers, and expectations that help will be forthcoming in certain areas only, must be added the inhibitions about self-disclosure:

Figure 1   Action systems and marital problems

Referral/presenting problem	Special features of the problem
(a) Couple acknowledge and seek help with marital problem	Couple may suffer from a range of material and emotional difficulties
	Suitable support may be lacking from agency to enable intensive therapeutic work to take place
(b) One or both parties seek separation	Worker may need to insist on initial conjoint work despite couple's or individual's insistence that marital relationship is over
(c) One partner referred, e.g. after attempted suicide	There may be little recognition of the marital problem initially, but readiness to involve other partner
	Emotional deprivation and social isolation of individuals make conjoint work unlikely to be initially possible
(d) Family referred because of problems with child(ren)	(i) child may be acting out difficulties between husband and wife
	(ii) Problems in family may reflect conflict or anxiety over parenting issues
	(iii) Either one or both partners may deny that family's problem arises from marital difficulty and tolerate intervention only if problem is located elsewhere in family

Goals of intervention	Targets of intervention	Action system
(i) Modify material difficulties	Relevant external agencies (e.g. DHSS, housing)	Agencies + social worker + couple
(ii) Clarify and resolve marital problems	Couple	Couple + social worker + on occasion other family members
To create physical facilities and supportive environment for therapeutic work	Social worker's own agency	Social worker + key members of management and team
Help couple and family work through issues of separation and disengagement	Marital dyad. May later become family and/or members of family as individuals	Couple + social worker. May later become family + social worker and/or individuals + social worker
Help couple resolve difficulties	Marital dyad	Couple + social worker + on occasion other family members
To establish trust and more secure sense of self through client/ worker relationship	Couple as individuals	Husband + worker. Wife + worker
After initial work with individuals Clarify and resolve marital problems	Marital dyad	Couple + worker
To take pressure off child and work with and resolve marital conflict	Marital dyad	Initially, couple + children + worker. Subsequently, couple + worker
To develop consistent handling and/or give reassurance over parent/ child relationship	Marital dyad	Couple + children + worker
To improve family functioning by alleviating marital problem	Marital dyad	Couple + children + worker

'In the area of marriage, it is clear that there are considerable
sanctions against disclosing to other people unpleasant aspects of
what is a highly privatised and encapsulating relationship.'

(Brannen 1980:468)

Problems such as lack of knowledge and information, or anxiety and
uncertainty surrounding the decision to seek or readiness to accept
help, may need to be matched by an equally acute unhappiness before
marital problems are acknowledged.

In addition to the difficulty of identifying marital problems and the
worker's own potential ambivalence about these, there is also the
common problem of how to shift the focus of work, and the client's own
ambivalence or resistance to this. As Tebboth (1981) has suggested,
recognition – i.e. involving the ability to identify cues given by the
client, and a sensitivity to what is being explicitly or implicitly stated,
however irrelevant it may appear to the presenting problem – is the
first important skill that needs to be developed. Without this ability to
hear as well as to listen, the social worker cannot reflect to the client
the cues that are being given in order to seek confirmation and clarification. This same skill is also essential in then helping the client to
embark on the painful process of explicit disclosure, and in giving
support and encouragement to the client in coping with the uncertainty and fears so often involved in facing up to a marital problem.

'Shifting the focus involves, paradoxically, staying where one is – at
least in the first stage. . . . The worker must be prepared to allow and
encourage the marital partners to explore and express their difficulty
without any immediate prospect of being able to do anything about
it. . . . If this is done successfully then it may be possible to offer more
formal, direct work with the marriage, with one partner alone, with
both partners separately, with both together, or even with the whole
family.'   (Tebboth 1981:13)

These constraints – worker anxiety and lack of confidence, organizational and statutory frameworks, and client inhibition – will have a
varying impact on the initial decision about focussing on marital problems, subsequent decisions about how to proceed, if at all, and the
whole process of intervention. The issues will affect agencies differently, but will revolve essentially upon questions of whether agency function and organization permit the focus, whether the clients can accept
and tolerate this, and how work should be conducted with the couple –
e.g. separately, conjointly, with the children or other members

of the family present, in a couples' group, or a mixture of these, and over what period of time and for what reasons.

Occasionally, although perhaps not frequently in non-specialist agencies, a couple may approach the agency seeking help with their relationship, having already identified this as problematic. In such circumstances it would be retrogressive to offer individual treatment, and it seems likely that many social workers would regard the marital relationship as the target and the action system. Decisions in these circumstances are likely to rest initially on whether the agency regards itself as having a statutory responsibility for offering such help. If it does, but fails to offer the organizational structure and support necessary to enable the workers to provide it, the social worker may need initially to make the agency itself the target for change. For example, procedures for the allocation of work, physical space within the building, and so on might be reorganized to allow social workers to sustain a series of regular appointments, whilst a support group of interested workers within the team might be organized or external consultancy arranged, with a view to providing continuing support and creating a climate in which such work becomes accepted.

In other situations the worker may decide that, whatever nominal responsibility the agency might have for such a referral, priorities make it unlikely that any extensive help could be offered. Very brief intervention – e.g. one or two interviews – might be offered in these circumstances, and the couple then referred to a specialist agency for further help.

If an offer of help is made, however, a decision is required about the appropriate action system to engage. Accepting the couple's own definition of their problem suggests that the couple should be seen alone for a number of sessions, for several reasons. First, the marital unit represents a discrete sub-system of the family system and the one that has sought help. To suggest involving the family system *ab initio* is unnecessary and may discourage the couple from pursuing the offer of help, especially if they feel their problems are private and that the presence of children or other family members would inhibit them.

Secondly, although the action sytem might subsequently need to be extended to include other family members, an informed discussion with the couple of the need for this will be difficult without a full appreciation of the problem. As Walrond-Skinner points out, however, it maybe appropriate to involve the children occasionally, 'if only to help the total family group to integrate changes that are taking place within the marriage' (1976:128). Equally, if one or both of the partners' difficulties involve conflicts with their families of origin, it may be important, where possible, to involve key members of the extended family. The principle underlying such decisions is one of including in the sessions those family members who are significant in the emotional transactions between the couple, so that the operative systems 'get worked with, not talked about, during sessions' (Walrond-Skinner 1976:128)

Thirdly, it must be recognized that there will be some couples who will gain susbstantial relief from counselling and the opportunity to discuss and reflect upon their thoughts and feelings about their difficulties. The involvement of the family in such a process would generally be inappropriate.

When the couple present themselves for help in this way, the action system of couple and workers should be modified only exceptionally. There may nevertheless be occasions on which it is appropriate to see each partner individually at some stage in the intervention process. Sometimes it becomes clear that one partner is too emotionally deprived to be able to share the worker and needs to be able to form a dependent relationship in order for any progress to be made; or one partner is involved in some situation, such as an extramarital relationship, that they are unready to divulge in conjoint sessions. In such circumstances the thrust of the work needs to be on the resumption of conjoint sessions, and the possibility of involving other colleagues in some way – e.g. to continue work with one partner on a one-to-one basis – may need to be considered.

A different kind of situation may present itself where the couple are struggling towards separation. Here the initial referral may come from one partner seeking help or perhaps hoping that their spouse will be persuaded to change their mind about leaving. Alternatively, as in some of the cases of attempted overdose described by Butler, Bow, and Gibbons (1978), one partner may be referred as a result of a crisis arising from the threat to end the marriage; or, as in Archer's (1982) case, one partner may already have left and be declaring that the marriage is ended. Assuming again that the agency accepts the referral, the action system that the worker should attempt to engage should include *both* partners and at some point the children too.

It is sometimes argued that where the goal of intervention is disengagement and the separation of members of the family, then individual work is indicated. However, in our view, the process of disengagement, the working through the sense of loss, the testing out of different ways of relating, and establishing a different sense of self are activities that need to be undertaken with and between all those involved. The particular action system engaged during the process should reflect the point reached by the disengagement. It may, for example, be appropriate to see the couple together initially, to explore issues of whether to separate, how to accept the fact of separation, and the issues of attachment and disengagement, followed by work with the couple and the children. An interesting extract in Gorrell Barnes (1984a) illustrates for example the way in which children can be helped, painfully, to explore the meaning to them of their mother's intended departure. Finally, by moving from conjoint to concurrent or collaborative sessions, or a combination of these, the format of the sessions will reflect 'the course of progressively decreasing intimacy which the couple is struggling to achieve' (Walrond-Skinner 1976:129).

In such situations, where the issues are fairly clearly about separation and the ending of the relationship, it may be important for the worker to be emphatic in opposing the way the client is inclined to present the problem rather than accepting and supporting this self-definition, as might be done in different circumstances. Unless the worker attempts at an early stage to do conjoint work with the marital dyad, the move towards separation will continue, possibly even reinforced by the worker's intervention with the couple as separate individuals, and the opportunity for conjoint work will be permanently lost. Thus the marital dyad should be regarded from the beginning as the target for change, and the action system the couple and one (or two) workers. This should be so even in those circumstances where one partner has sought help and continues to be 'the client' – i.e. in Pincus and Minahan's (1973) terminology, the 'expected beneficiary' at whose behest the work is carried out – throughout the intervention process. The target system may at a later stage be altered to that of the family system, and, at a later stage still, one or more members of the family as individuals.

In other situations, which are also not uncommon, one person may be referred and there may be little recognition or acknowledgement of a marital problem. Equally, the worker may feel that, however clear the evidence for marital difficulties is, the client may need to establish a relationship of trust before these can be broached. This might be indicated with highly defended individuals, for whom the disclosure of such personal and intimate matters would be difficult, or with very emotionally deprived and socially isolated couples. For such couples described by Mattinson and Sinclair (1979), the worker needed to become a reliable attachment figure and to work through the ambivalence that was the hallmark of their core sample of clients, before any agreement to discuss marital problems could be reached. In these situations it is helpful to regard either one or both of the couple individually as targets for change, and to accept the initial goal of treatment as establishing a more secure sense of self for the individual through the relationship with the worker (the initial action system). Conjoint work, the acceptance of the couple relationship as the action system, evolves at a later stage in intervention.

A further situation with which most social workers will be familiar is where one partner seeks help with a marital problem, but all attempts to engage the other partner prove fruitless. The dilemma then for the worker is whether it is possible to help one partner alone. There are considerable risks of making matters worse by doing so; the excluded (even though entirely self-excluded) partner may become increasingly resentful; some of the energy that could be going into the marriage may be syphoned off into the helping relationship; it is often difficult for the worker to avoid taking sides; and finally, it may be difficult to keep the focus firmly on the client, rather than slipping into inevitably speculative discussion about their partner, which may be fed back to them, usually increasing their resentment.

On the other hand, although some specialist agencies may have a policy of working only with couples, to refuse help to the partner seeking it seems unduly inflexible. Our preference, if attempts to engage the other partner fail, is to offer brief, time-limited intervention with a specific focus − e.g. to explore and evaluate the strengths and weaknesses of the marriage and to decide whether it contains enough that is positive for it to continue; or to discuss a particular problem in the marriage, focussing firmly on the feelings and reactions of the client. Thus, for example, in two sessions with a social worker, a woman suffering from low self-esteem apparently derived sufficient reassurance about her competence and general attractiveness as a person to return to her marriage with new confidence. Although it seemed clear that the husband (who refused to attend) was autocratic and undermined his wife, the social worker avoided discussing him and concentrated on helping the wife to identify her real achievements, and on examining her tendency to underestimate her own abilities. In such situations, the offer of time-limited help with an explicit purpose seems crucial in limiting the extent of the client−worker relationship and the potential risks of worsening the marital situation.

Finally, there are those situations, which are probably most numerous as far as non-specialist agencies are concerned, where there is involvement with a family because of difficulties either it or the community is experiencing with one of the children. A child may be battered or at risk; an adolescent girl may be staying out late and spending the night with older men; a child may be suspended from school and other siblings are reportedly beyond control; a boy is placed under supervision following a series of thefts; a two-year-old is admitted to hospital for failure to thrive; and so on. In such cases, where the agency's statutory duty to be involved is clear-cut, one or more members of the family may be expressing stress that may belong to the family system as a whole. Here it is usually helpful to hold an initial family interview for diagnostic purposes; this has the advantage of taking the heat off the 'identified patient', and of circumventing the tendency for decisions about the mode of intervention to be pre-empted by legal and bureaucratic processes that confirm the family's view about which of its members should receive treatment. It may be difficult, for example, for a probation officer to alter a family's expectation that the delinquent teenager, newly placed on probation, will be the subject of the officer's attention and support, if little attempt has been made during the court appearances to treat the behaviour as something in which all the family potentially are involved.

Social workers therefore need to make decisions about which part of the family to work with. These should be informed not only by an understanding of what the problem is about, but also by a recognition of the kind of constraint already discussed, which may influence the direction of the work undertaken. Even where the source of the family difficulty is located firmly with the marital dyad, who are therefore the target system, the couple's defensiveness about this may suggest that the family would be a more appropriate action system with which to work. In addition, organizational constraints or a particular clinical situation – e.g. a state of crisis – may further suggest a particular approach to intervention.

In deciding whether, other things being equal, the target system should be the individual, the marital dyad, the family system, or some other sub-system of the family, it may be helpful to distinguish between couple issues and parenting issues. The former might include, for example, those behaviours on the part of individuals within the family that reflect the unexpressed conflicts within the marriage and where 'the "married couple" is actually a triad because it is defined in terms of the inclusion or exclusion of someone else' (Haley 1976:151). The latter would include those behaviours that are more to do with conflicts about parenting, such as differing ideas about discipline or expectations of behaviour, or situations where the partner closely identifies and sides with one of the children, so that the boundaries between the marital system and the child become distorted.

This distinction between couple issues and parenting issues is of course over-simplified, but is useful in indicating when work should be primarily with one system rather than another. For example, in the situation of the adolescent girl mentioned above, she was acting out her mother's suppressed frustrations in the marriage; working with the marital dyad not only took the pressure off the girl but put the problem where it belonged. A young wife may batter her baby as the only way of expressing the misery she is experiencing in her marriage; working with the husband and wife conjointly about their differing expectations of married life recognizes the key operative system. In the cases described by Mainprice (1974), where the children are held to be expressing in their asthmatic conditions and persistent soiling the conflicts between their parents, the children's conditions improved as the therapist worked with their parents and made more explicit the problems between them. Or, in a case referred to a conciliation ser-vice for help in resolving constant friction over access, the source seemed to lie in the wife's refusal to acknowledge or accept the end of the marital relationship, and it seemed more productive therefore to focus initially on this than to attempt to set up better arrangements over the children.

Conversely, the difficulties experienced by one family known to an FSU were connected with inconsistencies in the way the parents handled the children. The arguments between the parents mainly concerned the way each responded to the children; and since the problems within the family system largely concerned parenting, it was felt appropriate, apart from one session in which these matters were discussed with the couple on their own, to work with the family system as a whole. In another case referred to a conciliation service, where the parents had been separated for some time and had managed the questions of custody and access quite successfully, conflict developed when the father remarried. This was principally a reflection of the mother's need for clarification and reassurance about the father's continuing involve-ment with the children, and the relationship between them as parents. A subsequent meeting with parents and children seemed crucial in allowing these issues, which affected all concerned, to be worked out.

Recognition of the nature of the conflict, and of what it may suggest in terms of a family or marital focus, is therefore an important criterion in selecting the mode of work. It is not the only criterion, however.

Walrond-Skinner points out that such decisions cannot 'be settled once and for all at the outset of treatment – since the dynamic, evolving character of the treatment process precludes any static solution' (1976:124). This may be particularly true when the choice is between the family and the marital system, since experience suggests first that the location of the problem may not be immediately clear from the diagnostic family interview, and second that work with the couple on their own may well not be immediately acceptable to them. In these circumstances it seems right – indeed, there is probably no alternative – to adopt the family as the action system, and to move into conjoint work with the couple when they are ready to accept this or seek it out (see, for an example of this, Skynner 1976:328 ff.).

There are two further dimensions of the decision: first, parents are often reluctant to discuss certain matters, particularly sexual ones, in front of the children, and this privacy should be respected just as, in fact, that of the children should be, and separate interviews offered; and second, children, with their directness and immediacy of expression, may often move things along at a pace that may or may not be helpful. Skynner found the sessions without the children a good deal less effective, and did not feel that there 'was really anything important that could not have been said in front of the children' (1976:340), particularly as later on the couple uninhibitedly discussed sexual matters in front of them. On the other hand, the conjoint marital sessions may have been crucial in confirming the boundary of the marital dyad, and perhaps in slowing the work to a pace with which the couple were more comfortable.

Finally, it may be necessary to maintain the family system as the action system throughout the intervention process, even though the marital dyad is seen as the target for change. Within some families, individuals may be so defended against acknowledgement of their difficulties, or have such fragile personality structures, that they can be prevailed upon to engage in treatment only if someone else in the family has clearly been identified as the problem or the reason for the meetings. In such situations it may be essential to maintain the family action system, and to work with the couple's difficulties within this structure. The reluctance of family members to relinquish their particular positions in the family, and the strategies that the worker must employ to allow the system to change, have been fully discussed by authors such as Minuchin (1974) and Walrond-Skinner (1976), who nevertheless underline the necessity on occasions of going with rather than opposing the family system.

Some of the issues concerning decisions about working with marital problems are illustrated in diagrammatic form in *Figure 1*. Having explored in this chapter some of the problems involved in identifying and deciding to work with marital problems, including the contributions of worker, agency, and client, and having outlined some of the factors that need to be considered in identifying the appropriate target for and point of intervention, we shall move on to consider some of the techniques appropriate for working with marital problems.

5

Operational concepts

There appears to be a growing acceptance of the need to distinguish between the knowledge required to understand a particular phenomenon or problem, and the knowledge required to try to resolve it. Fischer, for example, distinguishes between 'causal/developmental knowledge [which] focuses on answering the question "Why did a given state of affairs come about?"' and 'Intervention knowledge ... [which] is intended to be used to prescribe principles and procedures for inducing change in behaviours and/or situations' (1978:52). Thus, although understanding causation may be important in prescribing the areas and goals of intervention, it may do little to identify the actual techniques intervention may require. An explanatory view of the effects of maternal deprivation on the development of the personality, for example, may say nothing about what needs to be done in order to remedy the problems being currently experienced, these tools of intervention forming a distinct and additional body of knowledge with which the practitioner needs to be equipped. Chapter 3 therefore reviewed those explanatory concepts that are useful in understanding marital conflict, whilst this and the following chapter look at those concepts and models of intervention that may answer Fischer's second question about 'what can be done'.

There has also been a growing recognition that differences in understanding at an explanatory level are not necessarily reflected in intervention, and that practitioners from different theoretical backgrounds may in fact work with a case in a very similar way. Thus, in Chapter 3 couples' misperceptions and misunderstanding of each other were described as a common feature in the interaction of unhappy couples. Despite their different theoretical explanations for this phenomenon, therapists suggest similar techniques for intervention. Working from a psychoanalytic perspective, for example, Greenspan and Mannino (1974) suggest that the phenomenon of projective identification may be disrupted 'by the therapists repeatedly pointing out how the spouse differed from the projected image' (quoted in Segraves 1982:238). In other words, even though the explanation is in terms of object relations theory, at least one method of correcting the misperception could more accurately be said to be drawn from behavioural theories. Equally, behaviourists frequently augment their approach with techniques that emphasize the internal worlds of the spouses (e.g. Liberman 1975).

By grouping these techniques of practice together as 'operational concepts', rather than linking them to particular theoretical approaches, the commonalities of the approaches are emphasized. So too is the fact that although the thrust and direction of the work will vary depending on the practitioner's understanding of the case and the client's needs, the techniques employed in intervention may be drawn from a wide range of theories.

Because of the varying routes and settings through which help with marital problems may be sought and offered, it is difficult to identify a common starting point for the intervention process. Mattinson and Sinclair (1979), for example, describe the long period of contact that preceded a shared decision to work with the marital problems of their clients. In this chapter, some explicit or implicit agreement between worker and clients that work will focus on the relationship of the couple is assumed.

Establishing a working alliance

STRUCTURE

Joint or separate interviews   An early issue for the practitioner concerns the decision about working with partners separately but concurrently, or working with the couple together. The Institute of Marital Studies describe a method in which two practitioners work separately with the partners, joint interviews with all four participants taking place relatively infrequently. The understanding of the dynamics of the marital relationship is based primarily on the feelings that the client induces in the worker, since the clients will 'pull' the same reactions from their workers as they do from each other. Furthermore, they argue against seeing the couple jointly until each worker has established a clear picture of their particular client through the worker – client relationship, since without this, it is harder to perceive and understand the transference. As Guthrie and Mattinson argue,

> 'The transference of feeling to the worker is . . . usually heightened in a strong, one-to-one relationship, which the client feels he has for himself and which he does not have to share. His interaction with his partner can be more readily experienced by the worker in this situation. The number of clients per worker often reduces the invest-ment of feeling by the same amount . . . if the clients are not all using the worker as a recipient for the same feeling, they can distribute their emotions around, and then the worker, not feeling them himself, has to make a guess at what they are.'   (1971:57)

There are also certain disturbed clients who have such a small amount of trust that, although they can consolidate it within the tight confines of a one-to-one relationship and learn to generalize from this, involve-ment in a larger group would be experienced as overwhelming or threatening. Such couples can, however, make good use of a triadic exchange where work is with both partners together; and, in almost all other instances, this (or conjoint work with two workers) seems the preferred approach, for several reasons. First, the evidence suggests that marital work is more effective and progresses more rapidly when the couple are seen together (Gurman 1978). Second, experience shows that it is easier for both clients and worker to understand the relationship when it is enacted in front of the worker and all three can then stand back and examine what has taken place. In addition, whilst the value of the IMS approach to understanding and working with the transference is widely argued, the approach appears to many social workers to require inordinate skill and time. Third, as Chapter 3 argued, the concepts of projection and projective identification have yet to be validated empirically. Whilst the idea of shared binds is useful, there are many couples for whom either they do not exist or they are not a problem; and if they are there, they may be more easily recognized in a conjoint session.

Co-working   Although other forms of co-working may be useful (e.g. colleagues behind a screen, or concurrent one-to-one work with another member of the family by a co-worker), we are concerned here with the use of two workers simultaneously with the couple, and the potential advantages and disadvantages of this.

For many social workers embarking on work anticipated as complex and stressful, a co-worker provides reassurance, while shared discussions and observations after the session can prove an invaluable *aide-mémoire* and source of new insights. Co-working can also provide a useful way of sharing different tasks; e.g. it is often easier for one person to be involved in negotiations with the DHSS or writing court reports. Within the session itself, one worker may supply particular roles to which the other is paying less attention. Thus, a study of co-therapist behaviour (Dowling 1979) found that, although therapist style remained constant regardless of co-therapist or clients, therapists did vary the time spent on specific interventions according to with whom they were working. It is also possible for one worker to underline, clarify, or reinforce in other ways what the other has said, an activity that is harder to undertake working alone. Modelling is also usually accepted as an important function of co-working.

Co-working may also be useful when working with very deprived clients, or where one partner is very defended and needs more support and reassurance than one worker would be able to provide without skewing the intervention. In an account of work with a schizophrenic patient and his wife, Hamblin describes how,

> 'If the attention was given to one of them, the other reacted as though being killed . . . it became . . . acute in one interview when I was giving attention to Mr Weston and his wife reacted by becoming physically quite ill.'   (1970:10)

Although the client's attachment to the worker was crucial in enabling him to feel sufficiently secure to work on the marital relationship, the introduction of a co-worker might have eased the competition for the worker's attention.

However, although workers often instinctively select as a co-worker someone who complements their personal style, the tensions involved in marital work mean that unresolved conflicts between the workers may become apparent and be exploited by the client couple. The division of tasks suggested above may convey a message about relative power, or the relative goodness or badness of the workers, which plays into a common tendency on the part of those with marital problems towards splitting. Provided the co-workers are comfortable with each other, this may be usefully played back as a piece of reality-testing for the clients; but if it touches a particular uncertainty on the part of the workers, then it is harder to deal with openly. For example, a remark during conciliation by a father to the female conciliator in a male/female pair that 'she hasn't said much' was experienced momentarily by her as undermining; both conciliators quickly recognized, however, that this was an attempt on his part to ally himself with the male conciliator against the rather powerful women in his life. In a less open partnership, uncertainties engendered by the client's comment might have blocked a helpful response as the workers struggled to deal with their mutual feelings of rivalry or doubts about each other's effectiveness. In addition, as Walrond-Skinner (1976) suggests, the co-worker relationship may internalize the family problem, creating stress between the workers that demands resolution. This can then be reflected to the couple more vividly, however, having been thus experienced by the workers.

In marital work, co-workers need to guard against becoming too powerful, in a way that is perhaps less necessary in family therapy or group work, where co-working is often seen as a valuable bulwark against being sucked into a powerful system. At a simple level this may mean being careful about monopolizing or overwhelming a probably less articulate couple. At another level it may mean being sensitive to the kind of message conveyed by the co-workers, particularly if they are of opposite sexes, in terms of an idealized but unattainable relationship.

An important decision in co-working is whether to work with a colleague of the opposite sex. As we discussed in Chapter 4, this does have certain advantages in that it prevents the isolated member from feeling embattled as the sole representative of their sex. It may enable the workers to role-model certain marital and parental functions that are being discussed, to provide a potential ally in the opposite sex, and so on. Skynner (1976) describes working with his wife as a co-therapist, and suggests that this allows a greater freedom in discussing sexual relationships, or other matters whose discussion might normally be inhibited.

When working in pairs, sufficient time must always be allowed for preparation and discussion. Decisions need to be taken in advance about, for example, how to cover for absences or holidays, when work should in general continue with one worker; who will open, time-keep, and record the sessions; and how the workers will communicate with each other during the sessions. It may be helpful during the session to spend a few minutes in discussion outside the room, having explained at the outset that this might happen if the workers want to confer. Workers also must reflect honestly on their feelings about each other. If they are already conscious of irritations, or of being unable to discuss certain issues (e.g. sexual matters), then it is likely that these will be exacerbated rather than resolved in the course of a busy working week.

After the initial novice period, when a co-worker may provide invaluable support and encouragement, it should be possible to make judgements about when two workers are particularly indicated (e.g. with very deprived or disturbed clients) and weigh these against the known strengths and weaknesses of the co-worker teams available. It is, finally, worth bearing in mind that Rice, Fey, and Kepecs (1972) found that many practitioners, as they grew more experienced, came to value co-therapy less. There may also be pressures on the agency worker making co-working impracticable.

CONTRACTS AND SETTINGS

The likelihood of a somewhat ambiguous start to working on marital problems argues for the negotiation of a clear contract between the worker and clients about the work envisaged. This does not mean necessarily anything written formally, but that there should be some clarity about what is on offer, which should involve some statement about the intention to focus on the interaction between couples. Thus one couple, after an initial interview with the wife, were offered a series of meetings in order to see (picking up the wife's phrase) 'whether we can find ways of making you feel more comfortable together again'. A certain sense of delicacy about offering this focus is commonly experienced, possibly because the worker is reflecting the clients' feeling about the privacy of intimate relationships, or because of the worker's own feelings about this, or both.

Most social workers have also probably experienced the mixed feelings as the time for a difficult session approaches, the rather shaming feeling of relief when the clients do not keep the appointment, followed by disappointment when the implications of this sink in. Such feelings may be acute with marital work, with temptations to opt for doing something that is urgent and pressing rather than continuing the marital work, or not to make a further appointment immediately on returning from leave. Clients are also likely to experience mixed feelings and should be given the chance to discuss them. This shared ambivalence may be reduced if a commitment is made at the outset to an agreed series of regular meetings. Mattinson and Sinclair (1979) make the further point that this sets an important boundary of safety for clients who may themselves be struggling with fears of being taken over, or are working on the issues of dependency and attachment/ detachment, which are core couple issues.

An explicit agreement may also distinguish between what is currently being offered and what may have been offered before, either by a different worker or by the same worker in earlier contact with the couple. If such contact has involved a good deal of practical and material help, the indication of a different approach may help the clients to understand what this is, and may check the worker's flight into action. This is not to suggest that workers either would or should neglect practical problems, but that if these were the initial point of entry, a change of focus should be made clear to the couple. A separate appointment for dealing with other urgent problems may be appropriate, or, if the work is being undertaken with a co-worker, allocating specific tasks to one worker. A student and his supervisor, for example, were working conjointly with a couple when the wife was convicted of fraud; the student took the responsibility for preparing and presenting a court report, thus managing this particular problem separately.

The findings of Sainsbury (1975) and Brannen and Collard (1982) about what clients valued most in their social workers are worth bearing in mind in this context, suggesting the importance of an informal approach and the offer of time and commitment. The latter found that the situation that clients experienced as conducive to self-disclosure was one in which the worker was simultaneously friendly and sociable, impersonal and neutral, informal and with a lack of evident status differences, and both caring and trustworthy. The importance of these qualities may suggest that interviews in the clients' home are worth considering, although organizing this to ensure privacy may need some thought, and the potential value of a different setting – such as the worker's office – for exploring issues primarily associated with the domestic situation should not be forgotten.

GOALS AND TASKS FOR INITIAL INTERVIEWS

How work proceeds with the couple will depend partly on personal style and agency style, but particularly on what problems the clients present. In any event, certain initial tasks will generally need to be accomplished. Ideally, by the end of the first or second session, worker and clients should feel that there is a working alliance based on respect and trust on which work may proceed; the worker should have begun to develop some working hypotheses about the nature of the problems and their aetiology; and he or she should have begun to formulate some ideas about possible areas to work on and the most effective way of bringing about change (Segraves 1982).

Most couples come with feelings of anger, grievance, and hurt, and unless they feel these have been fully listened to, further work may be difficult. A key part in establishing a working alliance may therefore depend on each partner feeling that they have been properly heard and at least partially understood by the worker. In many instances, this process is in itself helpful, since one of the painful experiences in unhappy marriages is frustration at the lack of acknowledgement by the other of what seem legitimate grievances or concerns. The result of being able to state one's position and have it acknowledged by the worker (and possibly by the partner) is to feel less disqualified and perhaps marginally more in control of the relationship. This process may also, albeit temporarily, make the couple feel more in contact with each other.

In some instances, providing the opportunity to discuss and express feelings is sufficient to enable the couple to grasp it without difficulty. In others, the exchanges (or lack of them) are so angry, or so vague and confused, that the worker must intervene actively. For example, where a couple are at loggerheads, the worker may need to make some comment that sets aside the content of the argument and focuses on the partner's feelings about the issue in question, perhaps with a reflection of what the worker has understood the anger to be about. In one angry argument about a husband's apparent failure to collect his dole money, the worker-concerned commented to the wife:

'It's difficult to establish the truth about what actually happened as it was some time ago, and even if it had happened yesterday it might still be impossible. What I do hear you saying, though, is that it made you feel that you were the only one who could be relied on, and that every-thing in the family depended on you.'

In other words, where possible, accusations and blame of the other partner should be shifted into statements about the self.

With couples who find it hard to discuss or articulate, the worker may need to stay with these feelings, rather than push for some definite statement of the problem. Very often, one partner talks at length while the other remains totally silent, except for non-verbal signs of disagreement or withdrawal. Alternatively, both may apparently be in agreement that one is totally in the wrong or to blame. In these circum-stances the worker might offer to try to put the blamed (or silent) partner's case, as Haley (1971) suggests. It is important to be explicit about what one is doing, however, and in the process not to appear to take sides, although the pressures from both partners to do so should not be underestimated. For this reason, too, it is usually advisable to avoid premature attempts to clarify the role that one partner has played in the genesis of the discord, and to avoid interpretations about maladaptive behaviour, unless these can be directed at both partners. In fact at this early stage, because of the initially high anxiety level, and the importance of offering sufficient support and reassurance to both partners if they are to continue to be involved, it is better to concentrate on clarification and confirmation of feelings rather than interpretation. It is reasonable to assume (see Brannen and Collard 1982) that, despite the sometimes devastating lack of inhibition with which couples can attack each other, each feels a certain amount of shame at exposing their failures in front of another person or at facing the implication of the focus of work.

The knowledge of being observed, not only by a probably critical spouse but also by an outsider, may lead to attacks on the partner as a defensive manoeuvre against the more painful business of acknowledging one's own predicament and feelings. Reassurance and sincere confirmation of the areas where the couple are functioning successfully, or have done so in the past, are therefore more appropriate than confrontation or interpretation at this early stage in intervention. The important role of the worker in enabling the couple to face the difficulties they are experiencing must be emphasized. The worker's ability to accept and tolerate the expressions of hostility, worthlessness, and sadness not only provides fundamental reassurance, but can help the couple to accept more readily, within themselves and the marriage, negative or ambivalent feelings.

EXPLORING THE GENESIS OF DIFFICULTIES

A common dilemma for the worker in initial interviews is whether to undertake a detailed exploration of the history of the relationship. On the one hand, couples often feel the need to rehearse previous events, and to curtail this may be seen as a lack of interest or acceptance. The worker may also want to know how long-standing the difficulties are or whether they have been triggered by a particular event, and understanding past conflict may help this. On the other hand, the discussion can quickly escalate into unproductive recrimination about past failures, which can serve to reinforce the feelings of helplessness that are likely to be around. Therefore, when the discussion of past events ceases to facilitate clarification and exploration, it may be appropriate to acknowledge these feelings and to suggest that, since the discussion is aimed at finding happier ways of being together, it might be more profitable to switch focus to current issues.

During the process of developing an understanding of the couple's individual perspectives, the observed interaction will begin to suggest some tentative hypotheses about the underlying problems. Additional information will be gleaned from how they talk, the underlying themes of any abuse, and characteristic responses to the worker's interventions. This process of observation is often helped by encouraging the couple to communicate with each other as well as with the worker, which may encourage their normal interaction in the worker's presence. This will be discussed further in the next section. Useful though this may be, however, in enabling the worker to observe the couple's behaviour, some people feel uncomfortable addressing each other rather than the worker; and a direct request at this stage to talk to their partners, if they are not doing so naturally, may be inhibiting or produce a recrimination spiral with negative consequences. Since the worker's principal aims at this stage are to engage the couple in working on the problem and to formulate some tentative objectives, it may be enough to restate as clearly as possible the worker's understanding of the couple's individual perspectives on their problems, with some comment about the positive factors. The worker may then wish to suggest which areas to focus on in the next sessions, and possibly, although not necessarily, some relatively small shift in emphasis or mutual interaction for the couple to reflect and work on in the intervening period.

EVALUATION

It may see anomalous at first sight to discuss evaluation, which normally occurs at the conclusion of a process, in an opening section concerned with the initial stages of work with clients. However, the process and method of intervention cannot be discussed and contracts cannot be formulated without some consideration of outcome, the assessment of which requires some form of evaluation if informed decisions are to be made about the possible need for further work. Thus, what we are concerned with here is to consider ways in which social workers may begin to evaluate their interventions from the outset. Not only is it right that evaluation should become a normal part of the process of intervention, but such attempts by social workers themselves may increase work satisfaction as well as improve service to clients.

Space precludes a lengthy discussion of evaluation, which is an important subject in its own right. (For a fuller discussion, readers are referred to authors such as Fischer 1978, Jayratne and Levy 1979, Reid and Hanrahan 1981, Sheldon 1982 and 1983.) However, whilst much of the discussion concerning evaluation refers to the collection of quantitative data generated by the use of behavioural methods, it must not be assumed that evaluation is limited to such approaches. As Sheldon has argued, 'There is no good reason why qualitative data about changed thoughts and feelings cannot be gathered in as rigorous a way as possible' (1982:98–9).

One of the most straightforward and accessible approaches is that of single case evaluation. This offers an unpretentious means of evaluation that can be built into work with clients in an uncomplicated way, can be undertaken openly with them as a joint activity, and may provide a useful and concrete focus for work. It has advantages of providing both worker and client with direct feedback, which more formal research projects lack, of being responsive to the myriad of individual problems encountered, and of providing the worker with at least some information as to whether the help being offered is appropriate and successful.

The essential stages in using the single case evaluation method involve, first, clients and worker producing a clear definition of the problems, which should include an account of how it developed over time and what currently maintains it. Secondly, goals must be set that provide clear feedback in terms of enabling some measurement to be made of the progress of intervention. Thirdly, some intervention must be specified that it is hypothesized will affect the problem under review. This, as Baird (1978) points out, should be 'risky' in that it should be the kind of statement that can be confirmed or otherwise by subsequent events; e.g. if the couple are helped to talk through their disagreements, these will occur less frequently.

In formulating a general description of the problem, it is important to break down an abstract statement into specific components. Thus a statement that the wife feels unsupported must be explored so that the particular ways in which she feels isolated can be specified. These 'indicators' can then be used to monitor the presence and level of the problems and 'are usually key items of behaviour, or occurrences which reliably "stand for" and appear to co-vary with, the appearance of or the magnitude of the problem under review' (Sheldon 1983:483). For example, impressions about the extent to which a wife was feeling less isolated were 'anchored' by examining the extent to which decisions over spending money and the children's activities were taken jointly by husband and wife, rather than by the wife alone.

The next stage in the sequence is to assess the incidence of the problem experiences or behaviours prior to intervention – in other words to find a baseline from which subsequent improvement or deterioration may be assessed. Sheldon (1983) suggests various methods of developing baseline measures including direct observation, time sampling, participant observation, mechanical aids to observation, observation by mediators, and self-observation. Social worker and clients next have to decide what rates of behaviours would constitute an improvement in their particular case, 'remembering that sometimes it is not the behaviour *per se* that is the problem, but the rate or level at which it is performed, or the setting in which it occurs' (Sheldon 1983:486). They have also to agree a time scale for the intervention and the evaluation of outcomes.

Although there may be certain difficulties involved in this approach to case evaluation – e.g. in arriving at the appropriate specificity of the problems and measurements of change – we would concur with Sheldon that the general sequence that the method involves – i.e. formulation, hypothesis, intervention, evaluation, and follow-up – 'represents a considerable advance on the *ad hoc* procedures presently in use' (1983:499). It has the additional advantage of constraining social workers to be clear about their methods and objectives and of involving the clients closely with the change effort. It is also a method that readily complements some of the social-work approaches that we go on to discuss, and offers a manageable means of evaluating intervention as part of a process of continuous assessment and reassessment, thereby enhancing the ability of individual workers and the profession as a whole to demonstrate the effectiveness of intervention.

Working with the detail

It has long been a tradition in social work with a therapeutic aim to effect changes in functioning by focussing on pieces of behaviour, through which to promote larger shifts in critical emotional areas. This approach embodies a view of problem-solving behaviour suggesting that people deal with the minutiae of daily life in characteristic ways, which also reflect or are a part of their ways of dealing with larger emotional issues. By focussing on small sequences of interactive behaviour, highlighting and examining them, suggesting and trying out different ways of enacting them, and so on, the worker can attempt to alter a couple's transactions, thereby bringing about a shift that can be generalized to other areas of their lives. As William Blake expresses it in the poem *Jerusalem*, 'He who would do good to another must do so in Minute Particulars.' This section discusses some of the varied techniques involved in working with the 'minute particulars' of the marital relationship.

During the early stages of intervention, which are concerned with engaging the couple in work, forming some tentative hypotheses about their problems, and providing reassurance and confirmation of self, little attempt may have been made actively to promote change. The worker may even have curtailed the couple's exchanges in order to retain control and focus. Now, however, the workers needs to engage with the details of the interaction, a useful way into this being to facilitate the couple's behaving normally so that the problem can be observed as it were *in vivo*. The worker may choose to focus on some small non-verbal transaction that has been observed, or on a possibly trivial exchange the couple report having had on the way to the session, or on the style of their communication; where the sequence is highlighted depends on the worker, but in an important sense the couple have themselves identified the problem on which to work by discussing or enacting it in the first place.

With some couples there is no difficulty in eliciting couple behaviour, but with more withdrawn couples the worker may have to do more to elicit their characteristic interaction – e.g. suggesting that a comment made to the worker be redirected at the partner, or asking them to re-enact an argument that has developed during the previous week or to discuss in the worker's presence an issue that seems important to them. At other times, the worker can only deduce their interactive behaviour, perhaps from their mutual distance and from their similar response to the worker. One couple, for example, described an 'awful' evening that they had experienced the previous week, but seemed unable to say very much about it. The worker persuaded them to reconstruct the evening, asking them to recall their feelings. By commenting and guessing, the worker laboriously pieced the loose ends together, a process that left him feeling exhausted, as if he had been 'pouring energy into a leaking bucket'. This, and their non-confirming response to him, gave a fairly accurate idea of how they behaved towards each other as well.

WORKING WITH INTERACTING SENSITIVITIES AND PAIRED BINDS

One of the features that frequently becomes apparent from the re-enactment of the couple's characteristic behaviour is that they have developed ways of managing stresses in their relationship that in fact intensify the problems they are trying to resolve. Often they exhibit very similar or, at the other extreme, totally opposite interactional styles that react negatively on one another – e.g. mutual anger and criticism, mutual withdrawal, or withdrawal and pursuit where one partner's response of silence and withdrawal may intensify the other's need for discussion and contact, the pursuit of which may serve only to increase the other's withdrawal. These negative spirals frequently occur over issues to which couples share a special sensitivity, so that neither may feel sufficiently confident and free to comfort and reassure the other, responding instead by trying to resolve their own distress and thereby compounding their partner's.

Clients frequently describe situations or discuss them in a way that makes these interacting sensitivities clearly apparent. For example, one couple's respective sensitivities appeared to derive from earlier experiences. David anticipated and feared rejection, his mother having deserted him and his first wife having left him for another man. His anxiety resulted in bullying at any hint of his wife's withdrawing. Sue, with a domineering father and a violent first husband, reacted to the bullying by withdrawing, which David regarded as further indication of rejection. This pattern of interacting sensitivities was apparent in joint discussions, David questioning Sue peremptorily, Sue replying monosyllabically and distantly. This increased David's aggressive pursuit, such exchanges often ending with Sue making a remark such as, 'Oh what's it matter anyway?' and lapsing into complete silence. The worker was able to point out their mutual contributions to the transaction and how each was being deprived or provoked and instead addressed the underlying feelings of anxiety that prompted the unproductive sequence. Highlighting and interpreting the interaction, as opposed to commenting on the behaviour of one partner, underline joint responsibility for the relationship, and help the worker to avoid taking sides. This process also may enable each to recognize the feeling underlying the negative behaviour of the other – which, because of the need to marshal their individual defences to protect their particular vulnerability, may have hitherto been impossible.

REFRAMING

A useful technique in working with the detail of interaction is to attempt to shift the individual's perception and thus their experience of the behaviour or transaction. Watzlawick, Beavin, and Jackson, who called this re-labelling and redefining process 'reframing', define it as changing 'the conceptual and/or emotional setting in relation to which a situation is experienced' (1967:95). In reframing, therefore, the worker offers a different perspective on a particular situation, which, while fitting the facts, suggests to the clients a new and usually more benign way of regarding it. Thus, for example, the worker may suggest that although the wife is experiencing a husband's incessant questioning as nosey and intrusive, it can also be seen as an expression of care for her, which, although trying, may have a loving intent.

The frame offered to the couple may have an educative flavour, in that the perspective offered may suggest the normality of a particular dilemma and help them to feel less guilty or frightened by it. For example, a couple were experiencing sexual problems in their marriage and the wife was consumed with guilt and self-doubt over her feelings and behaviour. The worker commented that what she saw was a harassed, isolated mother of three small children, and she proceeded, by offering a different frame of reference in which the wife's unresponsiveness could be understood, to shift her client's perception.

As Gorrell Barnes (1984a) points out, this new perspective may be offered verbally, or may take the form of a task that gives permission or encourages the couple to see their dilemma in a new way. Such therapeutic tasks are considered further later; but as one example, a central difficulty within one marriage lay in the expression and management of feelings. The husband had an affectionate and outgoing personality but a rather clumsy and sometimes confused way of expressing himself. He was constantly wrong-footed by his intelligent but inhibited wife, who had a strong dislike of overt expressions of feeling and a preference for a quiet life, a situation reinforced by their somewhat reserved sons, so that the husband became increasingly isolated in the family. Reframing suggested that the expression of feelings was an essential part of family life, at which they both needed more practice, and the task between sessions was to practise engaging in vigorous and if necessary heated discussions about things that concerned them.

DISCRIMINATION TRAINING

A social worker may also attempt to correct the misperceptions frequently occurring between unhappy couples, by examining a piece of behaviour and demonstrating that it differs from the partners' perception of it. Thus the worker offers a different reality and draws their attention to the difference between their view of the behaviour and the partner's actual behaviour. The timing of this sort of intervention, which draws attention to discrepancies between perception and actuality, is critical, since it involves confronting the individual with a view of reality that may hitherto have been unacceptable. The following extract describes a couple who had already received some help in understanding and accepting their mutual difficulties about dependence and independence:

> 'On one occasion . . . Mr Armstrong reported what he felt was an improvement. They had arranged a family outing to the country and Mrs Armstrong was being her usual efficient self in preparing. . . . During this time she "rapped out orders" to Mr A, which always upset him. He felt she was implying how useless and unhelpful he was being. As they piled into the car, she turned to him briskly, saying, "Is there any petrol in the car?" He was about to blow up at what he felt was the final criticism of his inadequacy, when he noticed that her hands were trembling. He realised for the first time that she was not necessarily criticising him . . . [and] immediately felt differently and was concerned for her.'   (Mainprice 1974:46)

In another instance, the worker was suddenly struck, whilst listening to a wife's catalogue of woe that included a recurrent statement that her husband did not care for her, by an intense look of pain on the latter's face. She commented on this, saying that it seemed hardly the expression of someone who was uninvolved; the wife, catching the expression too, fell momentarily silent.

During such intervention, both partners may become increasingly anxious and unsettled and may struggle against the attempt to modify the interaction. It is not uncommon, in the middle of this process, for one partner to do something that almost seems an attempt to sabotage the whole therapeutic effort and to reassert the dysfunctional way of behaving. The worker then needs to intervene quickly to forestall the conflict starting again. Sometimes the contradictory behaviour is so blatant that it can be seen by all involved as almost comic, as in the situation where a wife started to read the cover of a magazine on the worker's shelf just as the latter was carefully pointing out her much greater involvement in her husband's concerns during the previous weeks. A long account in Minuchin (1974:178 ff.) also illustrates the painstaking nature of the technique, and a couple's resistance to changing perceptions. In this case, the husband is perceived as the sick partner, although the wife is also contributing to the problem. However, both partners, but the husband especially, resist the therapist's attempts to juxtapose a view of the wife's actual character and behaviour as possibly problematic with the husband's view of himself as the one who is sick and inadequate.

DEVELOPING A 'RELATIONSHIP ABOUT A RELATIONSHIP' (WILE 1981)

Watzlawick, Beavin, and Jackson (1967) cite a husband and wife who become involved in a bitter argument about an invitation that the former had issued to a friend, which perplexed them because both agreed that it had been right to invite him. They comment:

> 'in actual fact there were two issues involved in the dispute. One involved the appropriate course of action in a practical manner . . . the other concerned the relationship between the communicants – the question who had the right to take the initiative without consulting the other – and could not be so easily resolved digitally, for it presupposed the ability of the husband and wife to talk about their relationship.'   (Watzlawick, Beavin, and Jackson 1967:80)

They call such communication about the communication 'metacommunication'.

Much of what has been discussed in this chapter is concerned with metacommunication – helping couples to recognize what they say, how they say it, how they interact, and how to modify the 'rules' of these interactions. These strategies also have an overall purpose of helping the couple to observe their relationship, not only so that they might change it, but also so that they can at least recognize what they do without being overwhelmed by those aspects of their relationship that may seem distressing and intractable. For example, one couple were locked in a bitter fight about the wife's visit to her mother, when the wife broke off sadly and said, 'We're at it again. We'll just never agree on this', at which her husband also sighed and nodded. The worker said, 'Well, OK, perhaps you never will. But at the very least you know now more about why you can't agree – what it means to you both. And that disagreeing about this needn't mean you disagree about everything.' By developing this 'view of the relationship' – in this case by the wife recognizing that her husband's intemperate criticisms of her mother were partly an expression of his uncertainties about his wife's affections – they were able to understand the arguments and to contain and recover from them.

It may be argued that recognizing and understanding some conflict may begin to change it or, conversely, that recognizing something as unchangeable produces feelings of hopelessness and despair. Both may be true; change may gradually occur, and there is sadness in recognizing that a problem will continue. However, the recognition that 'this is what we do, how we behave' can be helpful in enabling people to feel more in control and less overwhelmed by the conflicts arising between them.

Working with communication

The review of explanatory concepts in Chapter 3 referred to the fact that both systems and behavioural theorists have regarded the ways in which couples communicate with each other as a key factor in generating and maintaining marital discord. Noller (1984) concludes from a review of the evidence that couples low in marital adjustment are more likely to misunderstand each other because of poor verbal or non-verbal communication. Although it would be simplistic to suggest that people's feelings can be resolved merely by tackling their communication patterns, or that communication problems can be isolated from other problems, it is also clear that couples get locked into unproductive battles and arguments, which only increase their sense of despair, because their feelings and opinions remain unheard or unheeded.

Giving couples feedback about their style and pattern of communication and suggestions about how to alter this can be helpful. It may give some relief, albeit only temporarily, from seemingly intractable conflict. It also gives the couple something tangible to work on and some reassurance that they can control what happens between them. Finally, the very experience of being listened to and observed by someone else may be helpful in heightening a couple's awareness of their interactions. Each couple's way of communicating is idiosyncratic, and the worker will need to listen intently for patterns, styles, or content to emerge that seem to trigger quarrels between the couple. There are nevertheless a number of common 'mistakes' that intimates make in communicating, familiarity with which is helpful in enabling the worker to identify them and to respond.

The principal task to be accomplished in working with communication problems is helping couples to avoid the turns and tricks of speech that trigger quarrels or prevent them talking issues through. A second task is to help them recognize that communication is a joint responsibility; messages should be conveyed as clearly as possible, and should also be listened to and clarification sought if the meaning is unclear. The emphasis on mutual responsibility often echoes work being done in other problem areas and thus reinforces an idea that is sometimes hard to convey. Thirdly, it should enable couples to begin to achieve greater specificity about their problems; these are often surprisingly hard for them to identify because of the conflict, which often results, for example, in an argument half-way through the discussion of an issue, which is then never completed. Finally, it is a means of helping the couple to have a 'relationship about their relationship', which was discussed in the previous section. Even if they cannot check themselves at the time, couples may be able to pinpoint retrospectively what leads to the escalation of the argument.

Many forms of unproductive communication can be observed (e.g. see Thomas, Walter, and O'Flaherty 1974), the following being the most common. Communication includes, of course, not only verbal statements but non-verbal signals, gestures, silences, and so on. As Watzalwick, Beavin, and Jackson pointed out, 'one cannot not communicate' (1967:49).

GENERALIZING COMPLAINTS

A common tendency is to accompany requests for change with a comment of the 'You never . . . ', 'You always . . . ' type. These are seldom productive since it is likely that all the listener's energy goes into defending their position; and, since exceptions to the generalization can usually be found, the request is lost in trying to prove or disprove it.

USING TRAIT NAMES

This also exacerbates conflict (although it may relieve immediate feelings), since the partner labelled as childish, a layabout, heartless, insensitive, stuck-up, or whatever will react only angrily or defensively. Identifying behaviour that is disliked and then suggesting modifications is more likely to be listened to by the other person.

DISCREPANT VERBAL AND NON-VERBAL MESSAGES

Usually this occurs when one partner verbally agrees to something while signalling by facial or bodily gesture anger or unwillingness to comply. Sometimes the worker can comment on the discrepancy — 'You looked pretty distressed when you said that' — or can turn to the other partner and say something like, 'Are you happy with that? Or would

you like to ask your wife more about her real opinion of the idea?'.
Noller's (1985) finding that non-verbal channels seem to be more open
to misunderstanding and the most frequently used to convey the
emotional significance of verbally neutral messages underlines the
importance of understanding and working with non-verbal communication.

TOPIC-CHANGING/GETTING SIDE-TRACKED

A frequent pattern between couples is changing the subject before the
first one has been talked through. This may take the form of one accusation being immediately countered by another on a different subject.
Not infrequently, the topic change occurs when the couple appear
near to agreeing on an issue. One partner changes the subject, often
to an emotionally loaded topic, and elicits a rapid counter-response.
The near agreement on the first topic is swiftly dissipated, the couple
being left feeling frustrated that nothing can be resolved. It is
important for the worker to maintain the original focus without alien-
ating the partner who has interrupted, perhaps by commenting on
the importance of the new issue and suggesting that it might be
returned to when the current issue has been resolved. Later on it may
be helpful to identify this side-tracking to the couple as problematic in
their interaction.

SEPARATING NEEDS AND EXPECTATIONS FROM UNFAVOURABLE
COMMENTS AND PUT-DOWNS

Couples frequently sabotage perfectly reasonable and acceptable
requests by attaching to them some complaint or thinly veiled criticism, thereby sending to the recipient a mixed message: a request for
change and an expression of disapproval or hostility. The motivation
for this is complex and may need clarifying before the communication
pattern is altered, but couples are often unaware of inviting rejection
by the nature of their statements and their failure to clarify why the
request is important to them. Inevitably it is to the negative content
that the recipient responds. For example, an exchange may begin,
neutrally, with a wife's request that the husband takes the children off
to the swings for a while 'because I need a break'. At this point the
wife's unexpressed feelings of harassment may lead to an oblique complaint, or one that the husband hears as anger against him – 'I've
had the children all day' – and immediately the husband may feel

defensive. Although initially, where anger may be intense, requests that are not accompanied by veiled hostility are hard to elicit, it may be helpful to emphasize that requests are more likely to be responded to if accompanied by positive signals.

PRESUMPTIVE ATTRIBUTION OR 'MIND-READING'

In Chapter 3 we discussed some couples' difficulties over closeness and differentness. Some writers (e.g. Satir 1967) have observed the tendency in the language of unhappy couples for the self—other differentiation to be obscured. Thomas (1977) labelled one facet of this 'presumptive attribution', where one spouse makes some assumption about the other's inner state, motivation, or feeling and then presents it as fact. The destructive assumption may be a hostile one — e.g. 'You only said that because you're angry at being alone over the weekend' — or it may be seemingly neutral but communicate to the partner some feeling of being patronized or taken over and be experienced as an assault on their autonomy.

USE OF FIRST PERSON PLURAL

Similarly, couples often use the first person plural and speak for both, thereby precluding open conflict or acknowledgement of differences. Since this may reflect a particular problem for the couple, it is sometimes appropriate to encourage more open disagreement by suggesting a greater use of 'I' statements.

INTERRUPTING AND NOT LISTENING

Couples frequently complain that their partners do not listen, which is often confirmed by the way they interrupt each other. Encouraging listening without interruption may enable them to complete discussions, which is one of the goals of working on communication difficulties. The worker must of course appreciate why the interruptions are occurring, since one partner may use greater verbal fluency (or verbosity) to dominate and control, making interruptions necessary.

Learning to express feelings more productively is implicit in many of these issues, but it may sometimes be appropriate to focus on this specifically, the objective being to encourage possible problem-solving solutions. A statement such as 'I feel A in situation B when you do C' does not attack the other partner's whole character and offers information that could help resolve the conflict. For example, 'I really feel disappointed when you don't come with us to Mum's for dinner – I wish you would' has more chance of being listened to and possibly acted upon than 'Why don't you ever come with us when we go to Mum's? You sit in front of the TV and never go anywhere', which leaves the other feeling attacked and unlikely to respond to the feelings being expressed.

Another technique frequently advocated by marital therapists is to suggest that the couple begin sentences with 'I', and try to avoid beginning them with 'you', which helps foster the expression and the acceptance of responsibility for needs and feelings. It may also make it harder to attack their partner, or to sustain the distortions of perception that may be included in the attack.

Given that communication is a two-way process, encouraging couples to listen and respond to each other effectively is equally important. Many workers adopt simple behavioural devices to foster greater awareness and responsiveness – e.g. encouraging couples to make eye-contact during a session, or to practise reflective listening by encouraging them to acknowledge what they have just heard, and stating what they understood of it. They may also be encouraged to give head-nods while one person is speaking or to express praise and approval as positive reinforcement to their partner. Feelings of being misunderstood and criticized may also arise when a partner is seeking only a sympathetic hearing to an expression of feelings, but the reply is limited to suggested solutions. As a result, the partner may feel angry or hopeless about the difficulty of expressing and sharing feelings. This may occur when a partner feels inadequate in coping with feelings and therefore responds with suggestions for action rather than responding to the feelings being expressed. In such situations the worker may indicate the nature of the desired feedback and that involved concern and sympathy may be all that is required.

Liberman (1980) suggests that couples may need direct instruction in giving praise or confirmation (which he calls 'giving pleases') and in seeking it and acknowledging 'pleases' when they are given, since both may assume wrongly that their partner really knows or should know what is wanted. Equally, habit and the anticipation of rejection may make the direct statement of requests difficult. The formulas and exercises he suggests may have a rather remote flavour, but they do underline the principle that sometimes style and habits of expression can be taught.

Communication patterns may reflect important underlying issues for the couple that may need to be addressed, or they may be considered almost in isolation as an example of faulty cognition. Thus, one client's swamping, mind-reading, interrupting style of communication seemed an accurate reflection of her internal state and of the underlying problem of dominance and weakness between the couple. The work with communication, to help her to make 'feeling-self' statements and to check her tendencies to 'mind-read', was one way of approaching the problem, but was carried on simultaneously with the worker helping her express and experience her feelings of doubt and uncertainty within the relationship. Alternatively, modification of one young couple's destructive quarrelling was the major focus of intervention, without any links or connections being made between their communication style and any underlying problems. Yet another couple, who were worked with over some time, seemed to experience some relief from their incessant arguments over trivia and to move closer to each other through developing more understanding of the mixed messages they were sending, although these were largely peripheral to their main problem of dwindling interest in each other. In other words, whilst working at the level of communication is a useful approach to work with couples, the extent to which this reflects other work being done on the same problem, or is offered as a temporary alleviation of conflict or as a solution to one problem among many, will vary according to the particular couple.

Changing behaviour through agreements

In one sense, there is something artificial in presenting a separate section on behavioural change, since many of the approaches for intervention discussed above are about helping couples through altering their patterns of behaviour. Thus, the examination with a couple of observed examples of their interaction may focus on behaviour that is a manifestation of inner states, with the aim of helping them change their relationship through altering such exchanges. However, marital therapists frequently find that couples identify behaviours not related to any inner state or problem that are a source of irritation, and agreeing to focus on and alter these can bring considerable relief. Similarly, it may sometimes be possible, having listened to a catalogue of complaints, to help a couple re-state these in terms that may then offer suggestions about how to alter behaviour. Moreover, couples can usually quickly grasp the ideas of reciprocity and positive and negative reinforcement, since they are close to their everyday experiences. Some straightforward explanation of these, and the generally greater effectiveness of positive encouragement rather than negative criticism, may be linked to observations concerning the couple's own mutually reinforcing patterns of behaviour.

As always, the question of timing is crucial, since trying to identify agreed areas for behavioural change will be difficult if the couple are totally at loggerheads. As argued earlier, therefore, it may be important to allow each considerable time to state their position and view of the history of the problem before either can 'inhabit the relationship' sufficiently to engage in this process. On the other hand, couples often despair of ever being able to alter things for the better, and some small but specific suggestion for change that can be agreed upon may be both reassuring and encouraging. In one instance, after a painful first session in which mutual accusations and recriminations had constantly flared up, the worker suggested that they needed to decide whether to hold the next session at his office or in their home again. The couple eventually agreed to have it at home, and the worker was able to point out that they had at least negotiated this together without coming to blows.

As argued in Chapter 3, a couple relationship is distinctive in that it involves a pattern of mutually reinforced behaviour. While the relationship continues, what one person does will impinge on the other and produce a reciprocal response. This must be remembered when helping a couple work out an agreement about behavioural change, since it may affect the kind of contract evolved. For example, one of the authors, working as a relatively inexperienced probation officer, helped a couple develop a contract on a tit-for-tat basis (sometimes called a quid pro quo), in which the husband agreed to escort their daughter (a school-refuser) to school, on condition that his wife had her ready in time. The husband's side of the agreement depended on the wife's performing her part, and when on the second day the child was not ready for school, the agreement fell apart. The disadvantage of this kind of agreement is that the behaviour desired by one is contingent on the behaviour desired by the other. One way of trying to circumvent this is to specify a period of time as the 'cycle' of the contract, after which the behaviour-changes should be resumed. Thus, in the above example, a new 'cycle' could have been specified to start the following day, so that non-performance of the tasks continued for only a limited period.

A different and less problematic kind of agreement is one in which the behaviours desired are not linked, each partner agreeing to perform certain behaviours in exchange for specified rewards, consisting of separate events. For example, a husband might agree to put the children to bed on certain nights each week, the reward being to be left in peace to watch sport on Saturday afternoons. The wife might agree to do the beds and empty the children's pots before her husband came home, and have an evening at bingo without being criticized for going out. Non-completion of either task would mean forgoing the reward.

The reinforcer in these agreements is usually chosen by the partner due to receive the reward, on condition that it is not aversive to the other partner and that it does not contribute to other problems. Thus, if the reward involves the other partner – e.g. where the husband desires a walk with his wife in return for doing the washing-up – it is important that walking is reasonably congenial to the wife, since if she dislikes walking, she is punished each time he washes up. Equally, the reinforcer should primarily reward the partner making the change, since something that rewards both also results in punishment for both if the desired behaviour does not take place.

In helping the couple to develop this kind of agreement, it is usually advisable to start with something relatively minor, since, at an early stage in work with the couple, bartering may not be concerned so much with changing behaviour as with the process – i.e. demonstrating symbolically that they are not powerless in the situation, and can act effectively and even collaboratively. It is unlikely, in the early stages, that couples would be ready to negotiate on highly charged issues, such as sexual behaviour, whilst doing so later on may be helped by some earlier experience of bartering about minor issues. Many people find the process rather artificial and even embarrassing initially and need encouraging to persist.

Eliciting possible 'barter-worthy' behaviours may require some skill and sensitivity on the worker's part. Couples are often at such a low ebb that they find difficulty in thinking of potential trade-offs or rewards; or the only behaviours desired may be highly charged, non-negotiable (e.g. the ending of an extra-marital relationship), or couched in very abstract terms. It may also be difficult to find behaviours regarded as roughly equivalent, and to ensure that the tasks are carried out with a reasonably good grace. One of the merits of the approach, however, particularly with couples in conflict, is that it largely avoids consideration of motive or intent; paradoxically, it may be easier to carry out certain tasks if there is no assumption that by doing so one is being loving or submissive. On the other hand, if the desired behaviour is 'greeting me when I come in from work', this is sabotaged if the greeting is given with a scowl, and it may be necessary to spell this out.

The agreements discussed so far are of a 'bartering' nature. Although they have an in-built lack of spontaneity, they can be effective in reducing the level of irritation or conflict and in developing the beginnings of collaboration. Often, however, a couple can identify a particular situation that is creating difficulties – e.g. conflicts arising because of the proximity resulting from a husband's redundancy – and can work out ways of behaving to make it more tolerable. With such arrangements rewards are unnecessary, which may prove a more comfortable negotiating process for both social worker and clients.

One criticism of such reciprocal agreements is that the effect of not fulfilling them can be discouraging for both clients and worker, and may lead to further antagonism if, for example, one partner has complied and the other has not. Clearly such a risk exists; if the effect of accomplishing something is encouraging, then not doing so may be discouraging. This risk can be limited by the worker not conveying too great an investment in the agreement itself but focussing on the 'how' of what may or may not have taken place rather than its success or failure. In other words, the behavioural change (or absence of change) is not seen as an end in itself, but as a means of achieving further understanding of the problem and the relationship. Equally, the task may be a success at one level but a failure at another. Thus:

> 'a partner who wanted 10 minutes of talking may discover that it is not the existence of talking but what is talked about that is important. The individual reading the paper [undisturbed] may learn that it is impossible to relax with the paper knowing that the partner is suppressing a wish to interrupt.'   (Wile 1981:184)

In such instances the task, although formally accomplished, could be seen as unsuccessful, since neither really enjoyed the requested behaviour, and productive at another level since it clarified some of the couple's feelings of loneliness on the one hand and of being hemmed in on the other.

Therapeutic tasks

Therapeutic tasks differ in an important sense from the kind of behavioural tasks described so far, in that they attempt some symbolic link between what is involved in the task and the features of the relationship that are being worked on. Three features are considered essential in constructing such tasks: first, they should have a clearly defined purpose within the plan of work and must be sensitively timed.

Second, they 'must be practised or tried out, either actually or symbolic-ally, within the therapy session itself' (Walrond-Skinner 1976:70). Third, they must be capable of being performed within the family out-side the session. For example, the aim of work with one couple was to create greater differentiation between them, to enable them to face and survive their disagreements and conflicts and to lessen their projection of this on to outside agencies. The 'therapeutic task' devised for them was for Mr G. to make a trip to the library on his own and choose a book of interest to himself but not his wife, while Mrs G. was to do the same after the next session. Much amusement was caused when Mr G. pro-duced a book on basketry, saying that his wife was all fingers and thumbs and would never be able to make canework, whereas he might.

Such home assignments are useful in much marital work. They encourage the social worker to be explicit with the couple about objec-tives, whilst giving the work focus and maintaining the impetus of the work between sessions. Also, when couples are edging towards a diffi-cult change, they may work at a problem, perhaps arriving at an under-standing of it or a conclusion, and then lose track of it when the intensity of the communication fades. The task may then serve as a concrete reminder of what was fleetingly understood. When the task is not accomplished between sessions, talking about this provides a way back into the problem and a means of exploring the couple's difficulty in transferring new behaviours and understanding into their everyday life. It may also be desirable sometimes to vary the timing of sessions – e.g. by increasing the gap between interviews to see if new behaviours can be maintained – and home assignments are useful in supporting these in the intervening period.

The use of a genogram

A particularly useful diagnostic and therapeutic device in working with couples is the genogram, which expresses diagrammatically family history and data across several generations. In addition to recording relatively straightforward data about marriages, divorces, remarriage, death, separation, the sex and birth order of siblings, and the details of more complex marital situations (e.g. children of different marriages), it is also possible to show diagrammatically relationships within families – e.g. close dyads, triangular relation-ships, distant relationships, and so on. A genogram therefore com-presses on to one page information that would otherwise require several pages of writing. More crucially however, it can vividly convey the kind of 'baggage' from the past which couples bring with them into their marriages and family life, and their experiences of such things as death, divorce, separation, rejection, and the likely impact that these will have on their expectations of relationships. Although the genogram can be used at any point during intervention (and may be usefully undertaken on one's own or with a colleague to gain further understanding of a case), it is particularly valuable in the early stages of helping: not only does it enable the worker to obtain essential information; it encourages the couple to move from a blaming or recriminatory stance, and takes the spotlight off the scapegoat or identified patient. It can also be important in clarifying expectations – e.g. clarifying that the worker is not there to adjudicate and that all will be involved in the process of finding solutions – and in avoiding the sense of going over the same ground again.

Genograms can be useful both with couples who are not very articulate and with those who are, since committing something to paper may enable them to 'see' things that months of talking might fail to reveal. This process of 'making the invisible more visible' (Gorrell Barnes 1984a:122) may be profoundly disturbing, however, and time may be needed for assimilation, whilst some clients may find the prospect of looking into their past too threatening. Any resistance should be respected, and the attempt to prepare a genogram either abandoned or left until the clients have greater familiarity and trust in the worker. Workers using this technique might usefully prepare their own family's genogram first, both as a way of familiarizing themselves with the method and of recognizing the kind of feeling aroused by it. A discussion of the drawing of a genogram together with an example (*Figure 2*) is given in some detail, since this may not be familiar or readily available to readers.

The central and primary relationship in the nuclear family – i.e. in marital work, that of the spouses – should be entered on the chart first, the ages of the partners in their respective symbols, and the date of their marriage or the start of their cohabitation on the horizontal line. The children of the family should then be entered, with the oldest on the left and their ages within their respective symbols. The genogram is then expanded to include each spouse's family of origin. Besides the details of marriages, separations, divorces, and deaths, it may be useful to indicate the physical location of the members of the family, since this may be an important indication of the cohesiveness and likely supportiveness of the family network. As the family is mapped out, it is important to discuss the individuals who are entered and to explore the functioning

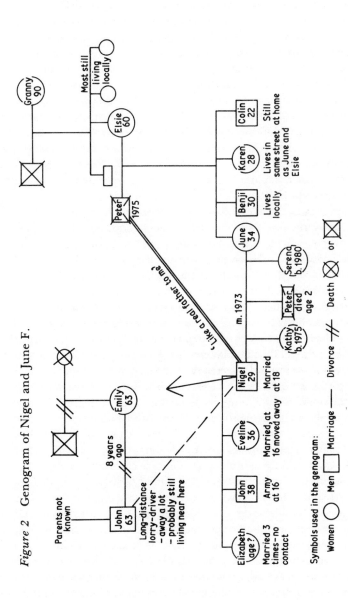

Figure 2 Genogram of Nigel and June F.

Symbols used in the genogram:

Women ◯   Men ☐   Marriage ——   Divorce —#—   Death ⊗ or ⊠

of the family, also including this information on the chart. For example, close relationships may be indicated by a thick line between the individuals concerned, affectionless relationships with a dotted line; if the relationship is imbalanced (for example, where a daughter seeks some affection from a rejecting father), this can be shown by an arrow in the appropriate direction over the line indicating the relationship. Any unusual information that is produced should also be written on the genogram – e.g. that the wife's mother was an invalid from the time the wife was eight, or that the father was away at sea or never stopped working. Since the chart may become crowded, it is useful to use different colours to indicate certain kinds of relationship or information. One spouse's family tree having been completed, the other's is then explored, if necessary on a separate sheet of paper, which should be placed adjacent to the first, so that similarities and differences in their respective experiences can be highlighted.

During the process of making the genogram, both the couple and the worker will often gain new knowledge and fresh insights into their experiences and relationship, which will suggest possible avenues for future work with the couple. In particular, the worker may be alerted to significant details or patterns that emerge within the couple's respective families. Facts previously unknown to either spouse or other members of the family, or not discussed for years – e.g. the birth of an illegitimate child, a miscarriage, or the absence of a parent during the spouse's childhood – may emerge. Some may have been forgotten, e.g. names or dates. Others may have an emotional significance, e.g. people may marry on their parents' wedding day, have died on their birthdays; or a child may bear the name of a significant adult and be seen as sharing their personal characteristics. Similarly, patterns may emerge – e.g. early deaths or particularly causes of death, divorces and remarriages, families with particularly large or small numbers of siblings, or sibling patterns that replicate each other with perhaps a wife being in a similar position in her family of origin as her mother was in hers, and so on. The physical and emotional closeness of the partners' respective families may also be significant – e.g. emotional conflict may be dealt with by becoming over-distant or over-involved – and their own experience of being parented should be discussed, since this will be relevant both to how they handle their own children, and also to what they expect from each other in terms of being parented.

In the example given, the lack of closeness and affection that the husband had experienced in his own family contrasted vividly with that of his wife's. Expressing it pictorially seemed to illuminate for them the mutual experiences that had drawn them together: she, the eldest daughter of affectionate but rather elderly parents, accustomed to looking after and protecting her younger siblings; he, seeking as he put it 'a warm lap to sit on' and unable to offer comfort when his wife needed to be supported after the death of their second child as an infant.

This chapter has explored a range of operational concepts demonstrating a variety of ways in which social workers can work with the detail of marital relationships once a working alliance has been established. These are not necessarily dependent upon specific theoretical perspectives or causal explanations. What is lacking, however, is a method or a framework for organizing the process of intervention and in which to apply these concepts, a task to which we turn our attention in the next chapter.

6

Approaches to intervention

This chapter discusses four approaches to practice that may be useful in guiding work with marital problems. Of these, crisis intervention, task-centred work, and group work are psychological in character, while sex therapy constitutes an approach to working on particular sexual tasks, using primarily behavioural techniques. This therefore appears after the section on task-centred work as a highly specific instance of that approach. Crisis intervention is discussed first, since work on marital relationships frequently begins because couples have exhausted their own resources and feel they are experiencing a crisis.

In Chapter 4, problems involved in the decision to work with the marital dyad were explored, with the suggestion that the systems approach devised by Pincus and Minahan (1973) might be useful in deciding when this should be the focus for change (the target system) and what network should be involved in bringing about changes in the marital dyad (the action system). In this chapter, although the target system remains throughout that of the marital relationship, the action system involved in each approach varies according to the particular dynamics of the problem and the approach to intervention that is adopted.

Crisis intervention

In many situations it may be appropriate initially to work with one or both partners who are in crisis, changing to a different approach when the crisis has abated. Butler, Bow, and Gibbons (1978), for example, first encountered the patients in their project after they had been admitted to hospital following an overdose and while they were in a state of crisis, and their initial work was concerned with helping the clients in the resolution of this.

The model hinges on the concept of crisis as an 'upset in a steady state' (Rapoport 1970) in which the individual's/family's/neighbourhood's customary strategies of coping prove inadequate, and for which new solutions are required. Crises are time-limited episodes, provoking a period of instability, which is gradually countered by the system's tendency to reduce disequilibrium to a tolerable level, after which the intensity of discomfort and motivation for change is reduced. How the crisis is experienced may determine whether the regained equilibrium is a positive or a restrictive adaptation to the changed situation. A primary assumption of the model is that dysfunctional adaptations to crises are not necessarily or even normally caused by prior failures in personality development, and that the successful resolution of a crisis depends on a number of contingent environmental factors at the point of crisis (Caplan 1961:186–87). Even where chronic damage to personality is evident, however, effective help can still be given. The emphasis is on the 'here and now' rather than on detailed exploration of past events, although the disequilibrium means that the client's defences are temporarily lowered and their feelings are more accessible, often enabling unresolved past conflicts to be dealt with.

A major difficulty with the model is the diversity of opinion about the definition of a 'crisis', sometimes including almost any significant event (e.g. McMasters 1957, Rapoport 1963), although there are certain characteristics of a crisis state over which there is general agreement. Crises are seen as being acute rather than chronic and are time-limited, existing for anything from a week to a maximum of about six to eight weeks. They are accompanied by marked changes in behaviour, in which the individual or couple are noticeably less effective than usual, and where much activity reflects an effort to discharge inner tensions, with a series of random and abortive attempts to resolve problems. The individual feels helpless and ineffective in the face of a threat to important goals, and may react with defensiveness, confusion, guilt, acute anxiety, self-pity and doubt, fear, and even anger and aggression. This is a particular possibility where a marriage is breaking down:

'each partner is part rejected, part rejector. Each is bound by remorse, pain, and residual love. Anger and cruelty set them free from these bonds: force their spouses to leave them, consume the stubborn stumps of their love, make guilt vanish . . . and from anger grows hate'   (Gathorne-Hardy 1981:171–74)

These reactions may be expressed also by physical tension and symptoms usually associated with anxiety, which may be a transitory response or a long-term adjustment to the crisis.

This then is the emotional context of the crisis. Both Murgatroyd and Woolfe (1982) and Jacobson (1983) have argued that, similar to the bereavement process, such responses follow a fairly well-defined pattern; the crucial difference between the two is that in bereavement there can be no uncertainty about the loss, but in marital breakdown there may initially be great uncertainty about the finality of the loss. This situation is further complicated by the fact that the lost person is still present in the physical world, and contact with them must be sustained at some level. None the less, although there are certain common crisis situations and responses, the individual's perception of what constitutes a crisis is unique, and one individual's crisis may not be another's.

The problem identified above in the loose definition of what constitutes a crisis may be overcome if a distinction is made between 'transitions', 'emergencies', and 'crises'. Transitions are events requiring the subject to expand the boundaries of their assumptive world, many of which will be desired and will be both anticipated and gradual. Emergencies are also encountered, involving loss and/or sadness but in which the individual may be able to rely on previous experience, or the event may be a calculated consequence of previous risk-taking decisions. Crises, however, are events in which loss and sadness predominate or are present in some measure, especially when the events leading up to them are sudden and unanticipated, and in which there is a fundamental challenge to the individual's assumptive world. As Getz et al. (1974) argue, the absence of a clearly distinguishable precipitating event is not in itself an indicator that a person is not in a state of crisis. Some people may feel reticent about divulging what has happened to them, and others may not know what led to their feeling overwhelmed or disorientated, but lack of awareness does not preclude effective intervention in the crisis.

An additional problem lies in the fact that a major life event such as marital breakdown may extend over much longer periods than the relatively short time periods referred to above. In order to resolve this theoretical and practical incongruity, Jacobson proposes the concept of the 'crisis matrix', which he describes as

'a period of several months to several years, during which an individual is particularly prone to experiencing several crises of the six-week type. Marital separation and divorce is such a crisis matrix.'   (1983:29)

In each of the crises in this matrix, individuals pass through at least two of the stages of crisis described below, although the third stage of consolidation would be unlikely to be reached.

The application of this model in practice may be more limited than it should be because social workers are not always available in crisis situations when intensive help is needed rapidly. A recognition of the importance of this could lead to increased accessibility; e.g. social workers could be based in job centres, housing departments, and similar 'front-line' agencies. In addition, although nobody is immune from crises, the stigma attached to social work may deter people from seeking such help. None the less, social workers in various settings do encounter people who are 'in crisis' as a result of marital difficulties and for whom an offer of immediate help can be of assistance. In the study by Butler, Bow, and Gibbons (1978), for example, of clients referred for psychiatric consultation, 83 per cent of all the married cases still living with a spouse reported a marital problem (Gibbons et al. 1979). Many of those referred to conciliation services soon after separation from their spouses are in a state of crisis. The emotional impact of marital breakdown is well documented (e.g. Ambrose, Harper, and Pemberton 1983, Belshaw and Strutt 1984, Hart 1976, Spanier and Thompson 1984, Wallerstein and Kelly 1980), and the extent to which it represents for many people a major crisis, which deepens as the relationship deteriorates and moves closer to final dissolution, has been graphically illustrated.

Social workers may also encounter clients in a state of crisis precipitated by some acute problem in the marital relationship, such as the discovery of infidelity or the sudden departure of their partner. Not all such crises, however, initially present themselves as resulting from some problem in the marital situation. For one couple, for example, the custodial sentence given to their son seemed to bring to the fore long-standing problems within the marital relationship, the wife being distressed at what she saw as her husband's callous behaviour over the sentence and his inability to offer her any support. Normally she denied these characteristics, but having been confronted with them and what they implied about their marriage, she found it intolerable to continue. Similarly, a husband's imprisonment may precipitate a crisis in an unstable marriage.

Crisis theory therefore offers a useful framework for working with certain marital problems, even though the precipitating factor may

be unrelated to these and may even remain unidentified. It is important to be able to recognize when someone is in a state of crisis and to
be familiar with the characteristic ways in which people in crisis display anxiety such as those suggested above. With marital problems a
more detailed diagnostic interview may be necessary than would normally be the case where the immediate nature of the crisis is more
readily apparent, as with bereavement.

A further feature of this model in relation to marital work is that, even
though the relationship is the target for change, the action system may
initially consist only of worker and one partner, with the involvement of
the second partner occurring as the work progresses (see Chapter 5). Or,
the crisis may have occurred because of the departure of one of the partners, and while an initial goal of intervention will usually be to engage
both, the initial action system again involves the worker and one partner. It is also not uncommon for there to be one person only who is
actually in a crisis state, and the concept of paired binds, where one person carries particular feelings within the relationship, helps to explain
this. In such situations the partner in crisis may be the client, the target
system the marital relationship, and the action system may be both
partners. An important goal here may be to enable both to experience
and share the anxiety about the marriage, thereby beginning to face
and cope jointly with some of the problems. An unfortunately unsuccessful piece of work illustrates this, in which a wife approached a social
services department because she could no longer cope with her husband's continuing blatant infidelity. They were seen together, and the
more the wife wept and pleaded, the more implacable the husband
became, denying that there was any real problem – 'it will only
threaten our marriage if you let it'. Four weeks of intensive contact saw
the wife move from abject despair to the point of carrying out constructive plans for leaving her husband, only after which did he seem
able to realize what was happening, and in his turn became despairing,
explaining that he 'had never meant it to come to this'.

Murgatroyd and Woolfe (1982) suggest a three-stage model that
may be helpful in understanding crisis reactions and in identifying
tasks for the worker in assisting their resolution. Although they discuss
the model specifically in relation to those experiencing the crisis of
separation and divorce, it is equally appropriate to those experiencing
other marital crises.

During the first stage of *orientation*, the person has to cope with the
changes in their emotional life that may be experienced as potentially
overwhelming and lead to high levels of stress, anxiety, and tension.

Typically, their response may be one of (a) denying that thoughts, feelings, or behaviour are altering significantly, (b) becoming or feeling helpless or depressed, or (c) seeking relief from tension through some outlet such as drinking, frantic sexual activity, or some precipitate action. Murgatroyd and Woolfe point out that although denial is likely to be a feature of this phase, individuals can cope either adaptively, seeking to minimize the stress without denying that it is present, or maladaptively, seeking to blot it out and deny its origins.

Crises in marriage are very often marked by the precipitate actions of one or both parties, and it may be important to help both parties to understand these for what they often are – desperate attempts to relieve the pain and tension of the current situation, rather than acts resulting from carefully thought-out intentions. Thus, when a wife left with her children to live with another man, without apparently giving her husband any warning of her intentions, it became clear that her feelings about her marriage were much more mixed than this apparently decisive action suggested. The worker helped them to see that this was neither necessarily 'bad' nor irrevocable, to work on the mutual feelings of despair that had precipitated the wife's departure, and eventually to agree to have another go at their marriage.

At this stage, the worker needs to convey warmth, reassurance, and concern. The ability to listen and respond sympathetically may be crucial to someone wrestling with feelings of worthlessness, a sense of failure, and possibly shame at being unable to cope. At the same time, the worker needs to gather enough information to build up a comprehensive picture of the crisis, the nature, extent, and history of this and previous crises, and the client's previous responses to these. Equally, there is a need to help the individual to reach an accurate understanding of the crisis, to see the interplay of the components of the problem, and to isolate specific sources of stress and unhappiness. The worker should encourage the client to focus on the crisis, denial being gently but persistently questioned, and accurate factual information being placed before them, if necessary repeatedly, until the full implications of what has happened sink in. Refusal to accept denial may be one of the hardest tasks for the worker, since it can appear unwarrantably intrusive or assertive. And yet this may be one of the real contributions that a professional worker as opposed to a friend can make, since the latter inevitably feels more constrained by the conventions of social behaviour.

At this stage, Murgatroyd and Woolfe suggest that the individual needs a model of self-care and respect. Real or symbolic gestures by the worker in offering help can be important in conveying the crucial message that the person is still valued. Having demonstrated their regard in direct ways, 'occasional but forceful reminders of the concern and respect felt by helpers serve both to encourage the person in distress and provide a model for the direct expression of feeling' (1982: 58). The worker's encouragement of this, and acceptance of anger, grief, frustration, and hopelessness, may provide real relief to the client.

Murgatroyd and Woolfe suggest that their second stage, *integration*, is characterized by a rather more balanced appraisal of the situation and that intensive worry work takes place around the question, 'Who am I?' Just as in the loss of bereavement, when it may be important to facilitate reminiscence of and reflection about the lost object, so in working with marital problems the crisis may induce deep feelings of loss of something precious and good. Equally, the crisis may involve a recognition, albeit subconsciously, that some change in functioning and behaviour is required; this, because it touches on the core of self, may induce feelings of sadness, helplessness, anxiety, or fear in response to the threat of change. The process of taking stock in order to begin to cope with the situation may also involve mourning for what once was, or was hoped for. Discussion of the reality of the loss may therefore help the person in crisis to move on to the next stage of making essential decisions and reorganizing their assumptive world.

Again, particular coping mechanisms are associated with this stage. Maladaptive responses are repression and depression. The period is often marked by a tendency to blame the other person as one means of warding off the need for personal change, and the worker needs to resist the temptation to collude with this, particularly as the boundary between offering support and sympathy, and being drawn into criticisms of the other partner, is difficult to maintain. One client, for example, when the worker consistently refused to agree with her criticisms of her husband, argued angrily that the worker must be either 'for her or against her'. Much of the work at this stage, which was possible because it was in the context of a very warm relationship, consisted of helping her to see that victim–persecutor relationships are rarely one-sided, and also that to continue to see herself solely as the wronged wife might be safe but was ultimately suffocating.

Adaptive responses, at this stage,

'involve the attempt to experience and work through the emotions and thoughts in such a way as to seek both to control them and to put them to use in the construction of an identity. "Mastery not misery is the essential aim."'

(Murgatroyd and Woolfe 1982:58–9)

To assist this process, the individual should be helped to identify irrational beliefs that may be held and change them so that they reflect more accurately the reality of the situation, thereby increasing their ability to cope. Other techniques may also be used: e.g. monodrama, in which chairs are used to represent other key people, and the person in crisis holds a discussion with them, playing all the parts himself; cognitive restructuring, where thoughts are made into more balanced 'here-and-now' statements, which can improve coping by identifying strengths and weaknesses; and self-contracting, where the individual makes an agreement with himself to change his thoughts or behaviour whenever 'negative' thoughts intrude (see Murgatroyd and Woolfe 1982: 139 ff. for a more detailed discussion).

In the final stage of *consolidation*, if it is reached, the process of intense worry-work and attempts to achieve mastery and new ways of coping with the difficulty produces a new determination and energy. At this point, the individual or couple may need help in renewing old relationships and developing new ones. A characteristic response to many crises is a period of withdrawal, and in the case of marital breakdown, or an act such as attempted suicide in the face of marital problems, people may feel embarrassed at what has happened and need support in making social contacts once more.

The point at which people are beginning to contemplate alternative ways of rebuilding their lives in the face of the crisis may therefore be the appropriate point at which to move on to the first stages of a task-centred approach, and to engage clients in the process of identifying problem areas to work on.

Task-centred work

Most social workers will be familiar with the principal tenets of this second model of time-limited work. A central assumption is that the effectiveness and efficiency of intervention may be considerably enhanced if efforts are concentrated on helping the client achieve specific and limited goals of their own choice within brief periods of intervention. The method aims to focus maximum worker and client effort in a limited section of the client's life, the client's motivation to resolve the problem being enhanced and maintained by setting time limits to the intervention from the outset.

The essential elements of the approach involve the selection of a target problem from the problems presented by the client, the use of tasks to work towards the alleviation of the target problem, and the negotiations between the worker and client as to the target problem, tasks, and time limits involved. As with crisis intervention, the target system remains the marital relationship, but the action system involved in intervention will vary according to the problem identified. If, for example, the target problem is defined as the couple's decision to separate, then the action system may involve one partner plus worker, either because of the other's unwillingness to be involved or because at a later stage this becomes appropriate, after the process of disengagement has been thoroughly worked through in joint sessions. Alternatively, where the marriage is under stess because of poor material conditions and this is identified as a target problem, the action system will involve external agencies in addition to one or both of the couple concerned.

Of particular relevance to working with marital problems is the fairly common finding that a longer period of time needs to be spent initially with the clients than is indicated by Reid and Epstein (1972). Experience suggests that two or more sessions may be required before it becomes possible to work on identifying the problem area. With clients who are still in a state of crisis, it is more helpful to think of early work as a form of crisis counselling, as discussed in the previous section, with the final stages involving work on selecting a target problem. Butler, Bow and Gibbons, for example, in commenting on distraught clients whose spouses have left home, say

'the client may then have to face the certainty that his or her spouse will not return. Coming to terms with this kind of knowledge takes time, and it is only when this process has begun that the target problem can be defined.' (1978:399)

Wise (1977), in using the model in a specialist agency, also proposes a longer period of initial work, in which a brief history of the marriage is obtained, during which process the client may be helped to recall and identify forgotten positive aspects of the relationship and of their personalities.

The process of engaging couples in work may also be lengthy when someone else in the family has been the original reason for the referral. The problem search in these circumstances may not begin until some willingness to become part of the client system and to engage in work has been expressed; or it may be a very painstaking process, in which the couple need help in formulating their inchoate feelings and anxieties into a clearer expression of what is wrong. Again, Butler, Bow, and Gibbons comment:

'Many problems are difficult for the client to define exactly, and helping the client to pinpoint the cause of these feelings can be a long process. It is a necessary process in that a hurried problem search may lead to the selection of an inappropriate target problem. Clients are often not able to put their problems into words clearly, and need to be helped to explore the dynamics of their situation before they are able to decide on their target problem.'

(1978:399)

A further modification that may also arise involves the operation of more flexible time limits than are suggested by Reid and Epstein. Although it seems appropriate to introduce the idea of a time limit during the initial contact, in practice it seems difficult at this stage for either social worker or client to predict realistically the length of time required. A helpful compromise is either to make a guess of the number of sessions, with an agreement to review this at a specified time, or to make the decision when tasks have been identified and a more realistic prediction is possible. A period of about three months from initial contact to the ending stages of work seems to approximate to most people's needs. Other issues that need to be discussed initially are the style of systematic work proposed, the setting for the interviews, and, most crucially, who is to be involved in these. Decisions about this may need to be postponed until discussions on the target problem are under way, but should at least be borne in mind at this stage.

Reid and Epstein (1972) describe the stages involved in the process of target selection as follows:

1 The array of problems with which the client appears to be concerned is elicited.
2 The different problems or different aspects of the problem are defined in explicit behavioural terms.
3 The problems are ranked into an order of priority according to where the major emphasis is placed by the client.
4 The target problem is tentatively determined in collaboration with the client.
5 The target problem is classified by the worker.

Clients sometimes have difficulty, however, in specifying what is troubling them beyond a generalized feeling of depression and anxiety; or, more often, they produce a long list of problems, and need to be reminded that this is only the first stage of the process of selecting one or two particular areas to be concentated on. Butler, Bow, and Gibbons (1978) suggest that difficulties over identifying the target problem often arise from uncertainty about the future of the marital relationship, and that for some people this may become the target problem, the task being the consideration of the pros and cons of various alternatives. They argue therefore that quite a lot of work needs to be done before the target problem can be selected:

> 'In order to work on marital problems it is essential for husband and wife to be able to come to some sort of agreement on the target problem, and to do this the social worker will need to help them listen to the other's perceptions and feelings.'
>
> (Butler, Bow, and Gibbons 1978:400)

During this period, some of the techniques that we suggested in Chapter 5 may appropriately be utilized, since part of this process of reaching an agreement may involve helping the couple to recast the problem into interactional terms. Wise (1977), for example, suggests that as the specific problem areas emerge, they need to be examined in terms of how they are a problem between the couple. Remembering that the problem area must be of the client's choosing, an important distinction must be made between asking about one partner's contribution to the problem or to the other's behaviour – in which case recasting the problem may be difficult – and asking the question, 'What are the problems caused *to the marriage* by this behaviour?' If, for example, one partner has a drink problem, this may be recast by asking the couple to consider 'the problems that this drinking behaviour causes in the marriage'. Reid and Epstein make it clear that although the problem task is of the client's choosing, this is arrived at only after a process of exploration and clarification, which does not mean necessarily that the problem should be accepted in the form in which the client initially presents it. None the less, delicacy and sensitivity are needed in describing the problem in a way that does justice to the client's perceptions of the predicament, but also offers some possibility for effective intervention. Some cases never get beyond this point in the process.

Having identified the target problem, the process of selecting the tasks through which to work is usually a briefer phase. Tasks may vary in specificity from, for example, the relatively general 'to show feelings more', to a detailed account of ways in which feelings should be expressed. The discussion in Chapter 5 about separating behaviour into manageable segments on which people can then begin to work is relevant here, and the suggestion that therapeutic tasks should be related to the dynamics of the clients' interaction should be borne in mind when the worker is helping the client to select tasks that can be accomplished and will achieve the ends intended. Although it may often be necessary for the worker to suggest tasks that might help, Butler, Bow, and Gibbons suggest that 'these are less effective than the initially more long drawn out process of getting the client to think out his own tasks' (1978:401). In addition, Reid (1975) indicates that tasks are carried out more successfully and target problem resolution is slightly enhanced when the social worker goes through a task-implementation sequence with the clients, including enhancing commitment to the task, spelling out exactly what should be done, exploring possible obstacles, and practising the tasks involved.

The tasks selected can be worked on both in the intervals between sessions and during the sessions themselves, particularly when tasks principally involve one client and worker. For example, a task for a partner trying to adjust to the breakdown of a marriage might be to explore and discuss feelings about this with the social worker. The failure to implement tasks sometimes suggests others that need to be added, or that the target problem needs to be redefined. One couple's failure to work on the agreed tasks seemed to occur because the wife became so exasperated at having to manage the children entirely on her own that at the end of the day she felt disinclined to co-operate in carrying out the tasks. Item 5 was then added to their task list to allow for this, thus:

1 Mrs W. to sit down and eat evening meal with Mr W.
2 Mr W. not to watch television during the meal unless jointly agreed.
3 Mrs W. to take and express more interest in Mr W.'s work and outside activities.
4 Mr W. to be more responsive to this.
5 Mr W. to look after the children for an hour before bedtime, or to put them to bed.

Finally, Butler, Bow, and Gibbons suggest that, because termination has been planned from the start, there may be fewer problems in coming to terms with this; and that where there are anxieties, it is possible to find ways of helping clients to cope with them. The final interview is the appropriate moment to review what has been accomplished, to explore future activities, to offer encouragement and praise for improvement, and to help clients recognize or voice negative emotions as well as positive feelings about what has been achieved.

Intervention in sexual problems

As we indicated at the beginning of this chapter, working with sexual problems can be viewed as a specific example of task-centred work using primarily behavioural concepts, which has developed its own extensive technical literature and methodology. It may therefore be helpful for social workers to approach it within the context of the task-centred model, and engage the client couple in the process of identifying the problem from which the target problems will be selected, one of which may be a sexual problem.

This is all the more appropriate because many sexual problems are related to broader difficulties in the relationship, and a problem search may in fact lead to the conclusion that the problem selected should be some other aspect of the relationship, with the expectation that working on this will alleviate the sexual problems without the specific use of sex therapy. The evidence discussed in Chapter 2 points to a close relationship between many sexual problems and more general difficulties in the marital relationship; a cooling in a couple's normal sexual relationship is frequently indicative of a troubled marriage, rather than the cause. As Belshaw and Strutt have expressed it,

'A regular sexual relationship with one partner touches deep aspects of our personality. . . . Like marriage itself, a healthy sexual relationship depends on a commitment which is continually renewed.'

(1984:58)

If the commitment to the marriage begins to weaken, the sexual relationship is likely to decline.

None the less, there are circumstances in which it is appropriate to focus specifically on sexual problems. During the process of discussing and identifying problems, it may become clear that sexual problems have become overwhelmingly important and that the couple wish to select them as the target problem. It may also happen, particularly in the early stages of marriage, that the problem may stem from ignorance of the physiology of sex, or from unrealistic expectations (see Polonsky and Nadelson 1984), and may be relatively easily remedied by discussion and information-giving. Other couples may find great difficulty in discussing sexuality, and it may then be appropriate to select a different target problem initially, moving to work on the sexual problem only when they feel more comfortable and familiar with the worker. Action systems may therefore include workers and individuals, couples, or groups, depending on the problem. The decision to work on sexual problems may also involve the alteration of an existing action system to enable the couple to discuss these particular problems more freely. Skynner (1976), for example, describes the way in which he moved, at the behest of the couple, from working with the whole family to working with husband and wife alone when they wished to discuss their sexual problems.

We referred in Chapter 1 to the liberalization of sexual attitudes and behaviour in recent decades, a process facilitated by the work of people such as Masters and Johnson (1966 and 1970), which also precipitated something of a revolution in the treatment of sexual problems. This has been most evident in medical settings and has resulted in a tendency for sexual problems to be 'medicalized', psychiatry in particular being concerned in the treatment of sexual problems, with social workers therefore regarding these as beyond their competence. Although some problems do need referral for specialist treatment, many difficulties may be alleviated by discussion with a sympathetic and sensitive worker. With some knowledge of the techniques involved, social workers can be effective in resolving sexual problems.

Although there is no single model, much sex therapy draws upon and develops the basic approach of Masters and Johnson and utilizes behavioural principles (e.g. Hawton 1985, Jehu 1979, Kilmann and Mills 1983, Leiblum and Pervin 1980). Clegg describes the marital sexual dysfunction work of the Marriage Guidance Council as

'a behavioural treatment . . . a brief, time-limited, directive therapy aimed at removal of the sexual symptom rather than at attainment of insight, uncovering of repressions, or resolution of unconscious conflict. . . . The focus of the work is on resolution of the sexual difficulty and *not* on other aspects of the relationship except in so much as they may be hindering work on the agreed areas of change.'
(1980:186−87)

Since this seems to represent the most commonly adopted approach, a brief enumeration of such methods of working with both individuals and couples in relation to the main groups of sexual dysfunction is appropriate, although others (e.g. Dickes 1984, Dicks 1967, Tunnadine 1970) describe a more psychodynamically orientated approach, whilst yet others (e.g. Barbach 1980, Burbank 1976, Kilmann and Mills 1983) have argued the merits of group-work methods. A more detailed description of both the dysfunctions and the techniques described, most of which can be practised by the couple as 'homework' assignments, may be obtained from Hawton (1985) and similar publications.

It is important to understand something of the etiology of sexual problems before embarking on work in this area. Nadelson (1983) has defined three basic groups of sexual dysfunction symptoms:

(a) Those with a primarily organic origin, such as biochemical or physiological disorders, specific infections or tumours, anatomical problems, post-surgical problems, and various neurological, vascular, and endocrine disorders. In this context, drugs (prescribed or otherwise) and alcohol may be significant. Relatively common disorders such as arteriosclerosis, arthritis, diabetes, epilepsy, hypertension, multiple sclerosis, and renal disorders can all have varying effects on sexual drive and performance (see Hawton 1985:75–94).

(b) Those with a primarily psychogenic origin, which may stem from well-established intra-psychic factors, or from situational or interpersonal disturbances. As Nadelson has argued,

'Since sexual responses are a complex of autonomically mediated reflexes the person who is relaxed, not distracted, and well functioning psychologically is likely to be more sexually responsive. To function well sexually, the person must be able to abandon him/herself to erotic experiences and give up control, and some degree of cognitive contact, with his/her environment.'   (1983:15)

(c) Those whose origins lie in a combination of (a) and (b). Such problems, which are both complex and frequent, might include problems emerging after an acute illness, such as a heart attack, or an injury, which may call for a change in technique or in the pattern of sexual activity. Similarly, since both self-image and body-image are important components in sexual functioning, physical changes due to ageing or as the result of surgery – e.g. a mastectomy – may also lead to reduced sexuality and therefore to changes in sexual behaviour that may be seen as problematic.

It is also important to distinguish between primary dysfunctional syndromes, in which the problem has always existed, and secondary syndromes, where performance has been satisfactory but has recently become problematic. Nadelson comments that the former 'are more difficult to treat, and the progress is less optimistic, since the etiology is often more complex and undetermined, and congenital organic factors may play a more prominent role.'   (1983:20)

A detailed assessment and history-taking is therefore an essential prerequisite of any decision about the nature and scope of intervention (see Hawton 1985). This may be undertaken jointly by male and female therapists, although Watson (1984) argues that single-worker assessment is more economical and as effective. However, the process must involve both partners; we share with Watson the basic assumption that 'in every case of sexual difficulty arising between two people, the relationship between the partners requires assessment' (1984:58).

It is also widely accepted that couples often request help with a sexual problem when it is apparent that there are serious underlying relationship problems, which may well limit the success of any treatment focussed solely on the sexual problem (Clegg 1980, Nadelson 1983, Watson 1984). It is important to consider this during the process of identifying the target problem, since the worker's sense of the futility of embarking on work with the sexual problem may conflict with the couple's urgent desire to do so. Although there are no easy answers to this, for the worker to embark on a form of treatment that seems doomed to failure appears as hazardous as for the couple to be over-persuaded in selecting a target to which they feel uncommitted.

Whilst the detail and extent of the assessment process will vary with the nature of the problem, issues such as early sexual training and experience, family and personal attitudes towards sex and displays of affection, and their place within the marriage are important areas for discussion. Of central relevance is the chronology of the experience of the problems and their association with external events or triggers, whilst the possible significance of alcohol and drugs must not be overlooked. Watson (1984) also argues that, since client motivation is of central importance in determining outcome, some assessment of commitment to working on the problems is important, perhaps through some form of 'homework' before the next appointment – e.g. the completion of a questionnaire by *both* partners concerning sexual and medical history. It is only on the basis of a thorough assessment therefore that decisions about the possible need for medical examination and treatment, or about the nature and focus of appropriate social-work intervention, can be made.

Nadelson (1983) identifies certain basic principles of sex therapy:

1 The responsibility for treatment should be shared by both partners, who may also both be expected to share in the treatment process, so that it is clear that neither is the 'sick' one in need of treatment.

2 The social worker must provide an atmosphere of optimism in which sexuality is accepted, sexual enjoyment is encouraged, and support, help, and encouragement are provided. One potential difficulty that may need to be overcome is the worker's own diffidence in discussing sexual problems, since it is essential that embarrassment, surprise, or adverse reactions to descriptions of sexual attitudes or practices are avoided.

3 Enjoyment of sex rather than performance and achievement should be stressed, thus reducing the emphasis on the achievement of orgasm every time sexual activity occurs.

4 Both physical and verbal communication are important and may even be the primary focus, in order to achieve mutual understanding of attitudes, values, needs, and preferences.

Specific verbal or even written contracts may be helpful. As Gullick (1983) argues, whilst these should be flexible, they should also be clear, dealing only with observable behaviours, and be as positive as possible. They should be aimed at increasing positive behaviours rather than reducing negative ones and be as simple as possible, perhaps even being limited to one or two behavioural requests per partner.

There are certain problems that arise specifically in men or in women, and these we now consider.

MALE PROBLEMS

Impotence   Primary impotence or erectile failure is rare, but secondary impotence, as a response to illness, personal crisis, or other marital and family problems, is more common. Individual therapy is unlikely to be helpful since the problem is often a result of specific external factors, or of anxieties specific to sexual situations. Explorations of these anxieties through discussion may be helpful, in conjunction with specific techniques to be practised at home with the partner, aimed at focussing attention on genital sensation through caressing (both genital and non-genital), perhaps using lotions and erotic fantasies, moving on to masturbation once the man is having erections. Before intercourse is finally attempted, the 'waxing and waning' technique can be used further to reduce anxiety associated with loss of erection. This involves the partner ceasing stimulation once a man has a strong erection and allowing the erection to subside for a few minutes before resuming caressing. This can be repeated several times during a homework session.

Premature ejaculation The extent to which ejaculation is premature is partly determined by the responsiveness of the partner. Repeated failures may lead to secondary impotence or anorgasmia in the partner, which may be the presenting problem, so a detailed sexual history may be essential. Of central importance is teaching that control is possible, even in a state of intense sexual excitement. The techniques now available make this problem relatively easy to manage. The man must again focus on the genital sensation of his partner's caresses, learning to identify the point after which ejaculation is inevitable, at which point his partner ceases to caress him. After a short time, when his arousal has subsided, this process is repeated three or four times. This 'stop-start' technique can be used in conjunction with the 'squeeze' technique, in which the partner squeezes the head of the penis between thumb and first two fingers for 15 to 20 seconds, just prior to ejaculation. Both techniques are most easily practised with the man lying on his back and his partner alongside, or on top between his legs.

Retarded ejaculation Retardation or failure in ejaculation is usually situational. This fact can be established by the man masturbating on his own. The man should again lie on his back and focus on the genital sensations of his partner stimulating his penis, perhaps using a lotion or a sensitizing jelly. The degree of stimulation should be increased over several sessions, leading to ejaculation near the vaginal entrance and eventually in the vagina itself. At this stage, it may be helpful for the man to lie on top since this often facilitates ejaculation. Retarded ejaculation may also be found in younger and less sexually experienced men and may be associated with rigid and compulsive personalities or feelings of guilt. Concurrent discussion of such feelings and attitudes may also be helpful in such cases.

FEMALE PROBLEMS

Inhibited sexual desire This results in a lack of the normal physiological responses to stimulation, with the result that intercourse may be difficult. It may be intra-psychic or interpersonal in origin, and therapy may well focus on resolving general relationship issues. Inadequate foreplay or negative attitudes towards sexual behaviour and arousal may come to light. Exercises to develop and control the muscles surrounding the entrance to the vagina and the pelvic floor (known as Kegel exercises), often recommended before and after childbirth, may be helpful here. The exercises involve clenching and then releasing the muscles of the sphincter, as if to prevent and then allow urination. Women may be instructed to develop control by practising this while urinating. The muscles should be contracted initially at least three times as firmly as possible, three times a day, gradually building up to ten contractions at a time (Hawton 1985:218–19). Such exercises should be used in conjunction with sensate focus exercises, both non-genital and then genital, accompanied by sexual fantasies. Erotic literature may also be a helpful stimulus.

Orgasmic dysfunction   A woman may be sexually responsive but fail to reach orgasm when aroused. This is likely to be associated with cultural or psychological factors and may involve fear or anxiety about loss of control, total giving, or unrealistic expectations. If primary total orgasmic dysfunction is involved, a masturbation training programme for use by the woman alone may be relevant. Once orgasm has been experienced, genital sensate focus exercises should be used, the woman showing her partner how she likes to be caressed, leading eventually to intercourse, perhaps in conjunction with clitoral stimulation.

Vaginismus   Vaginismus is the involuntary contraction of the outer vaginal muscles, making intercourse painful or even impossible. Treatment is aimed at helping the woman to become more familiar with and accepting of her genitals through self-examination and the gradual introduction of different forms of vaginal penetration. Muscular control through the use of Kegel exercises may also be useful, in order to learn to relax. The process of gradual genital exploration and penetration should then be repeated by the partner in the context of caressing and pleasuring sessions. The process is one of gradual desensitization, although difficult cases may require clinical treatment.

Dyspareunia   Dyspareunia, or pain associated with intercourse, may be organically or psychologically based, and the treatment is similar to vaginismus. The main goal of therapy is to help the woman to enjoy sexual contact and to become sexually aroused. Different positions for intercourse, which avoid deep penetration, and exercises to increase the focus on genital sensations are the main elements of treatment.

Although a good basic knowledge of sexual physiology and responses is essential, as Hawton argues

> 'An important advantage of the current therapeutic approaches to sexual problems is that, by and large, they do not require an exhaustive training in a particular specialist field.'   (1985:4)

Such approaches are readily usable by social workers, who are thus much better placed and qualified to work with sexual problems than is often thought. This is particularly so since many problems have a psychological basis and may be amenable to a range of interventions currently practised by social workers, in addition to the specific sex-therapy techniques outlined above. Simultaneous intervention with either situational or interpersonal factors may be appropriate, particularly since clinical evidence shows that the number of people who can be treated with a specific behavioural approach alone is limited, and that a combination of approaches may be called for.

There are also, of course, specific sexual problems relating to ageing, physical handicap, and victims of sexual assault, and those relating to gender identity and sexual deviance. These are too complex to be discussed here, however, and are not frequent in their occurrence as marital problems.

Using groups as a medium for helping couples

Although we do not underestimate the obstacles involved in setting up groups for couples in non-specialist agencies, their potential therapeutic value for helping distressed couples is considerable. Small groups offer unique opportunities for experiencing reassurance, a lessening in feelings of isolation through sharing experiences with others with similar difficulties, and learning through modelling, social comparison, feedback from others, and testing out new interactive behaviours. In a review of the effectiveness of couples' groups, Gurman concludes that among other things the group experience 'facilitated the clarification of self-perception and perception of the marital partner' (1975a: 198) and a lessening of the ambiguity and uncertainty around marital role expectations, because of a greater readiness to express negative feelings towards partners in a non-threatening therapeutic setting. Groups may therefore be particularly effective as a means of working with mutual misperceptions, which are a common problem in marital difficulties.

Some discussion concerning the setting up and running of such groups is appropriate. It may be helpful to explore the key features of this approach, although the reader is referred elsewhere for a more detailed discussion of these (Heap 1977 and 1979, Whitaker 1976 and 1985). When using groups the potential action system, consisting of workers and three or more couples, is self-evident, although decisions about membership and size are rather more complex.

SELECTION AND COMPOSITION

Skynner (1976) suggests that, in contrast to groups of strangers, less attention needs to be paid to selecting couples. A wide range of personality, problem, and degree of disturbance seems possible because each participant is a member of a pair, and the possibility of becoming isolated – at least in the early stages – is therefore minimal. It seems likely in relation to couples' groups, however, that including couples *and* single partners may lead to conflicting goals and purposes, and that homogeneity of affective disposition in groups – e.g. levels of inhibition, depression, or extroversion – may lead to difficulties. By contrast, diversity of age, life-stage, marital experience, and marital difficulty are often felt to bring positive benefits in working with couples (Skynner 1976). Young couples, for example, may revive memories in older couples of the positive aspects of their earlier life together, and so on. On the whole, the greater the diversity of the group, the more protracted will be the initial stages in establishing trust and facilitative norms within the group, although this will also be influenced by the urgency of need experienced by group members. Where the inhibitions in expressing problems are considerable, as they may well be in marital work, then it is important to schedule enough meetings – e.g. a minimum of fourteen – to allow for a fairly slow initial phase.

Not everyone will benefit from being in a group, and exploratory interviews with potential members provide a means of assessing the likely benefits and costs to them of joining a group. For example, a client may be experiencing a crisis unique to him, or one that demands more immediate attention than a group may provide; or he may be too vulnerable to tolerate a group experience (see Whitaker 1985: 172–75). Interviews are also essential in explaining to potential members the purpose of the group, since many groups flounder because of members' confusion about this, and an important first stage in developing a consensus about this occurs even before the group meets. A statement of intent by the leader orientates potential members to the group, provides a realistic basis on which to decide about participation, and provides the group leader with some gauge of the threshold that the client has reached. In working with couples, where there may be uncertainty about readiness to acknowledge marital problems, there does seem to be a temptation to obscure the objectives of the group. For example, the leaders of a group for parents of adolescents recently placed on probation discussed its aim with two couples, who seemed a long way from recognizing that their own marital problems were a major source of difficulty for the children, in terms of issues of parenting difficult children. However, two other couples and the group leaders felt that marital difficulties should be the principal focus for discussions, and the group therefore started with two rather different agendas, which were never fully reconciled.

SIZE AND CONSTANCY

Most writers agree that for groups aimed at personal change, the optimum membership is 6 to 8. This is big enough to generate the kind of action – e.g. modelling, or revealing alternative experiences and solutions – that is needed therapeutically, but small enough to prevent any members drifting to the periphery, creating a split between core members and spectators. In a group where considerable confidence and trust must be established to enable members to risk discussing intimate matters, constancy of membership is important. Careful preparatory work, and the setting of a time limit on the duration of the group may often help to forestall dropping out or irregular attendance.

DURATION

Short-term groups limited to 6 to 8 sessions are common in social work. Whilst this may be appropriate for some groups (e.g. people in transition, such as prisoners about to be discharged), therapeutic groups require time in order for the necessary trust-building to take place. Decisions about the duration of a group must depend upon the personalities and problems of the group members, but for a couples' group a period of at least four months may be appropriate.

CO-LEADERSHIP

Certain features of groups – in particular the complexity and rapidity of the exchanges that occur in them – argue strongly for sharing the leadership with someone else, especially when couples are treated in groups. This view is to some extent supported by the available research evidence; Gurman, for example, concludes that 'tentative evidence suggests that co-therapist teams may be of special value when couples are treated in groups' (1975b:423). Co-working may offer particular advantages to social workers who are inexperienced in running groups, and who may feel some anxiety about broaching certain subjects with couples. In addition, the exchanges in couples' groups have an emotional intensity that can at times be overwhelming, and a colleague may supply much-needed support and assistance. Skynner (1976) goes further in suggesting that two therapists of the opposite sex offer additional advantages through modelling, which besides providing support and mutual aid is an important source of learning. However, although there are some advantages in this, co-workers of opposite sexes can offer a spurious model and may be confusing for leaders and members alike. In these circumstances, co-leaders need to do a great deal of preparatory work themselves in exploring their relationship with each other and discussing their prospective roles within the group.

LEADERSHIP ROLES AND TASKS

A leader can enter a group by several routes — e.g. taking over an existing group, or coming in as a consultant — which will affect the way in which leadership tasks are undertaken. However leaders enter, they are never the only source of leadership in a group. The leader is inevitably embedded in a leadership pattern in which members also assume certain leadership functions. None the less, although some leadership tasks may be distributed throughout the group, the designated leader retains special responsibilities and tasks — i.e. structuring, maintaining, monitoring, and intervening.

Structuring The leaders must have a clear idea of the goals of the group, and communicate these both before the group begins and in the initial group meeting. Although the leaders need to describe the point of the group as they see it, the goals must be worked out mutually and re-explored as the group continues. Thus it might be sufficient for leaders to confine introductory remarks to a statement such as, 'The group is intended to help members understand and work on problems being experienced in their marriages', and some reiteration of the duration of the group, length of meetings, and so on. The extent to which ground rules are introduced in the opening sessions

will vary; some leaders make statements about, for example, expectations as to confidentiality, penalties for non-attendance, and contact
with leaders outside group sessions. Our preference is to keep these to
a minimum, largely because it is easier to work problems out in a
specific context rather than to legislate in advance for something over
which leaders may have little control.

Maintaining   The way in which liaison with other workers who are
involved with group members, or with other professionals, is carried
out needs to be agreed between leaders and colleagues. Decisions
about the type of recording must be taken, bearing in mind the different purposes of a group record – e.g. sharing information with other
workers about individual members, keeping track of events, and
reflecting on conduct of groups. One can anticipate that significant
life events may occur for group members, and broad decisions about
how such events should be handled need to be taken in advance.

Monitoring   Groups are so complex that most people prefer to operate in terms of some conceptual framework that enables them to interpret events. There are a number of frameworks available (e.g. Brown
1979, Douglas 1979), but the model of group focal conflict seems the
most coherent and helpful for this kind of therapeutic group. It suggests that, at times in a group, a wish, impulse, or hope may emerge –
e.g. the wish to be closer to others – that is shared by the members of
the group (the 'disturbing motive' in the language of the model). This
is often accompanied by a related feeling of guilt or fear (the 'reactive
motive') – e.g. the fear of being rejected. These shared wishes and
fears constitute the group focal conflict. In an effort to deal with this
conflict, the group may adopt a way of behaving (a 'restrictive' solution') – e.g. mutual denial, blaming someone else, taking turns to
speak – that precludes both the exploration of these fears and the
expression or satisfaction of the wish. In contrast, an 'enabling solution' – e.g. acknowledging that everyone present has faults or that
feelings of anger or envy are universal – deals with the fear whilst also
allowing expression of the wish, so that 'wider explorations' are possible (see Whitaker 1985: 45–59 for a more detailed discussion). In using
this framework, it is important to try to listen at the individual level, the
interpersonal level, and the group level. An additional factor in
couples' groups is that each couple has its own history, because of which
and their interpersonal relationship they are members of the group.
Much can be learned about the dynamics of their relationship

from observing their individual interactions with other group members.

Intervening   Anything that a leader says or does in a group, whether a non-verbal gesture of support, encouragement, or disapproval, or a statement, question, or interpretation, constitutes intervention. It is difficult to summarize briefly all the numerous ways in which leaders may intervene, but it may be helpful as a way of underpinning various styles of leadership, first, if leaders see themselves as doing what appropriately belongs to their role as leaders – e.g. opening and closing meetings, structuring, preparing the group for termination, managing the boundary between the group and the agency – and, secondly, that they should do what no one else can do or is doing – i.e. supplying the missing roles in the group. For example, this might involve supporting and encouraging the development of a facilitating atmosphere; or alternatively, the group members may be highly supportive and reassuring to one another, and it may then rest with the leader to test the reality of the consensus, or to suggest an alternative way of looking at a particular issue (the 'reframing' discussed in Chapter 5). Skynner argues that therapists need to be 'prepared to intervene much more forcibly and directively than is usually necessary in ordinary stranger groups' (1976:255), and this may be seen as supplying a control role that may be missing because of the potential in couples' groups for destructive or aggressive behaviour.

There are also certain types of intervention that, although not exclusively the province of the designated leaders, more frequently need to be made by them. Members often adopt a shared defensive style of interacting as a 'restrictive solution' – e.g. talking endlessly about trivia, taking turns in speaking, or colluding in placing one person in a special position or role. This protects them from discussing issues that are painful or difficult. In these situations, it is usually only the group leaders who can break through the defensive pattern. Assuming that the group contract is clear, that the members know what they are there to discuss, and that the early exploratory stages are passed (when it may be necessary to 'test the water' by talking about unimportant issues); then leaders may need to intervene to break through the collusive defence.

For example, a group may have adopted the restrictive solution of being excessively polite to each other, and one might guess from this that fear of retaliation is leading them to suppress anger or disagreement. The leaders may then demonstrate, perhaps by openly disagreeing with each other, that disagreements are allowed and can be survived. Or one leader may give a 'read-out' of what has been observed, such as, 'I've noticed that people are very polite to each other and I wonder why that is', or 'Sometimes people feel it's important to be polite because they are afraid of what might happen if they aren't.' Usually if the group is ready to relinquish this particular defensive interaction, one member will then take up the leader's comment in a way that opens up the discussion. Thus, in a group for married couples where one spouse was physically handicapped, the leader realized that the group had already met for five sessions without mentioning problems of sex, which she guessed were around. 'Permission' to discuss these was given obliquely by telling the group the story of a paraplegic man, whose wife went to their GP to ask for the Pill and found that the GP was quite amazed that she needed this as he had imagined their sex life had ended with the onset of the handicap. Following this, after a short pause, the group sprang to life, sharing experiences and fears about sex.

Group leaders may also find that they may occasionally need to make brief interventions that may be described as instructing. In small helping groups where an important part of the learning is accomplished through feedback and support, the leader may need to teach the group members how to offer this in a way that is helpful and usable. In an attempt to be supportive, members may make global or generalized statements, such as, 'Your real problem is your mother-in-law', or 'Your trouble is you're shy.' The leader may then have to intervene somewhat directively, explaining that people are most helped to master a problem by being able to talk it through and make sense of it themselves. Or, whereas comments about what 'really' are the problems may be inappropriate, observations about how they experience each other within the group are appropriate and can be helpfully fed back.

Finally, in following the individual's experience in the group, leaders may sometimes wish to ensure that a particular experience or transaction in the group has registered. This may involve pointing out a non-verbal event – e.g. in the group described above, one couple had been addressing the group rather than each other as they expressed their doubts about their continuing relationship, but by the end of the discussion had moved visibly closer together – or a verbal exchange that in the leader's view is crucial, the implications of which are in danger of being lost because of the rapidity with which groups move. For example, in a group where a husband's inability to express his feelings had been the subject of much discussion, the leader used a pause in the group to underline the fact that the husband has just expressed himself quite aggressively and no one, including the husband, had been damaged by this.

In a short account, it is possible only to highlight the main issues to be considered in running groups for couples. We believe, however, that groups are under-used in working with marital problems and that, although there may be difficulties in establishing such groups in non-specialist social-work settings, once started many of the problems that beset other helping groups – e.g. devising an appropriate programme of activity, or the unwillingness of members to discuss important problems – do not occur, and they can provide a valuable and satisfying context for therapeutic work.

Conclusion

We suggested in our opening discussion that it may be appropriate to use crisis intervention in early work with couples, and then to move to a task-centred approach after the initial crisis has abated. Depending upon initial and subsequent assessments, it may in fact be appropriate to use the major forms of intervention discussed in this chapter sequentially, moving from an action system that involves the couple, or the couple with their children or external agencies, to one that includes other couples in the same predicament, as and when the circumstances and the dynamics of the problem suggest this should be done.

7
Marital problems and ethnicity

Some of the difficulties of identifying and working with marital problems amongst ethnic minorities were referred to in Chapter 2. As Roger Ballard has observed,

> 'Although there are now substantial Asian and West Indian settlements in most major British cities, the issues which their presence raises for the social services are still being approached with uncertainty.'   (1979:147)

Khan (1979) has argued that, unless there is some appreciation of the changes that migrant parents have experienced and of the attitudes that they have brought with them to the provision of help, the services cannot begin to know how to explain effectively the use and workings of their personnel and provisions. Therefore, 'In times of crisis, many people turn to friends, family or kin before considering the relevant statutory service' (Khan 1979: 2).

The relative under-use of various services by immigrants and their descendants is often assumed to be because problems, be they emotional or practical, can be dealt with by the family. Marett, however, in a study of Ugandan Asians resettled in Leicester during the 1970s, found that a need was being expressed for some form of 'counselling' help with a range of problems, including marital problems:

> 'Whatever their expectations of such a service, there was an assumed common factor: the helping agency was envisaged as outside their immediate family group, or even people within their own community.'   (1983:540)

Atma (1985) also argues that there is a need for such services.

A major problem in responding to such requests for help lies in the assumptions that are too readily made on the basis of too little knowledge, resulting too often in a process of negative cultural stereotyping. As Ahmed has argued, for example,

> 'the Afro-Caribbean family is often seen as a tangle of pathology, virtually non-existent as a unit or rapidly falling apart, with mothers too strong and fathers abrogating responsibility. On the other hand, the Asian family is often seen as problematic because roles are rigidly defined, with the mother's position weak and the father's authority all too pervasive.'   (1983:22)

Roger Ballard (1979) has indicated that it would be wrong to assume, if an Indian or Pakistani woman is in conflict with her husband, that the traditional subordination of South Asian women to their husbands or the institution of the arranged marriage is necessarily the source of the difficulty. Whilst such a view may be partially correct, such role relationships and institutions are central to the organization of South Asian family life, and it is unlikely that the wife would wish to alter her situation in any fundamental way.

It is therefore important to look beyond such cultural stereotypes and to recognize, for example, that although Asian women may appear subordinate, in reality they often have a great deal of authority and strength, having learned very early on in family life how to achieve their own aims. In such joint family systems, each individual is fighting for some power, including the mother-in-law, the son, and the son's wife with the other women. Whilst such struggles may not be readily apparent to an outsider, they are clearly recognized by everyone within the family. Social workers need to be aware of such processes when responding to requests for help from individuals who are part of such a system (see Atma 1985).

It must also be acknowledged that, in many westernized families, the system of arranged marriages is being combined with western marriage ideals, thereby allowing the couple who are to marry to meet and get to know each other, with the result that love marriages are becoming fairly common. Many Asian women, however, still accept the system of arranged marriages, and to know under what system a marriage has been arranged is therefore important. Amongst Muslims, marriages are arranged between close relatives – first or second cousins; uncles and nieces – and the parents themselves may be cousins. The advantage of these marriages is that all the members of the family know each other well, and the couple have a lot of time in which to become aware of their parents' expectations. If the idea of marrying a particular cousin is abhorrent, there is time to change and refuse, which many do. On the other hand, when this type of couple are in marital dispute, the whole family are involved and need the social worker's help. Because relationships are so intimate, the feuding can be bitter and painful, often extending back a couple of generations, sometimes involving relatives in other countries, and splitting the family. Social workers unfamiliar with this kind of situation may find the quarrels petty and too involved, whilst also feeling apprehensive about their ability to work in such situations.

A Muslim couple with marital problems illustrate such a situation. They had four sons, the husband was in a good job, and both he and his wife stated in court their desire for a reconciliation and that the dispute was between other members of the family. The wife insisted, however, that they should live separately from the family, especially his mother, whilst the husband felt unable to buy a house without his mother's approval. The husband attended counselling sessions with his mother, who tended to cancel whatever agreements he made with his wife. She in turn attended with her brothers, one of whom, to make matters more complicated, was married to her husband's sister. The resulting conflict split the entire extended family into two camps. The National Marriage Guidance Council Asian Counselling Project in Bradford (Atma 1985, Mitchell 1984) has been established to assess the needs of Asian families for help with marital problems and to develop appropriate services and training approaches. The Project has found that it receives many similar referrals from families who have exhausted the avenues of the family and the community, and who have reached the stage where they feel the need for outside help.

Amongst Indian families, however, marriages are arranged through a negotiator or an intermediary, often through the newspaper columns. Since for many families in Britain 'suitable' partners – i.e. from the right caste – are not available in this country, the partner often has to be 'imported', which presents its own problems. Whichever partner is 'imported', there may well be feelings of isolation and vulnerability, of being alone. When conflict arises in such marriages, it can be due to a number of causes over and beyond a difference of opinion between the couple. The groom's negotiator or advertisment may have been less than honest; he may have some handicap, not be educated, not have the job he said he had, or he may have been previously married and have children. The family may also begin to find fault with the bride — with her dowry, her looks, or her education. Unique problems can also arise in such marriages, the nature of which may not be immediately apparent. Thus a young Sikh wife, married about two years, sought help because her husband was not supporting her and their thirteen-month-old son financially, their only food being provided by the father-in-law. In addition, her three sisters-in-law were trying to get rid of her. In spite of these problems, she was reluctant to leave since she had no extended family of her own in this country. Discussion eventually revealed that her marriage had been arranged whilst she was in India, by her uncle during a visit to Britain. Within a week of the marriage, her husband's mother, who had brought about the marriage, had died, and he had reverted to living as a bachelor since he no longer felt the same obligations.

An awareness of and sensitivity to cultural issues is therefore clearly important in working with problems involving arranged marriages. It is equally important to recognize that significant changes have occurred amongst many communities (Atma 1985), particularly during the last decade, the reasons for which are manifold. Amongst some Asian communities, for example, a major factor is that many of the men who emigrated to work in British mills and factories are now unemployed. Consequently, women have become increasingly aware of their rights as they have learned how to use the British welfare system. In the past, women who were in conflict with their husbands were frequently dependent on help from their male relatives and were often persuaded to remain with their husband even if he was violent, since they were reluctant to return to their maternal or parental homes and become a burden on their families of origin. Such women may now seek help since, although they may be illiterate, they are aware of their rights and that they now have the option of leaving their husbands and becoming independent.

In spite of such changes, it is essential that social workers sensitize themselves to these complex background cultural issues, perhaps through some of the accounts of life in local immigrant communities (e.g. Singh, 1980) that attempt to unfold the realities of life for ethnic minorities in Britain, both at a community and at an intrapersonal level, as well as broader studies (e.g. Cheetham *et al.* 1981). Cross-cultural contacts in social work are nevertheless inherently problematic. Clients' identities are often firmly rooted in a cultural background with norms and values that are totally alien to the social worker, whose own background, norms, and values may be equally alien to the client. Similarly, the social worker's view of the world is 'culturally biased and may include both conscious and unconscious elements of prejudice. Thus social workers, through self-examination, must identify how their own cultural experience may contribute to possible prejudices.'

(British Association of Social Workers 1982:64)

Roger Ballard found that

'many people had learned only to present a fraction of their real concerns, for they did not *expect* outsiders to have any understanding of, or sympathy with, their own customs and beliefs. Indeed, a frequent strategy was to present problems in a way which, they hoped, would make sense in terms of majority assumptions.'

(1979:153)

This view is echoed by Marett (1981), who suggests that, even after several decades of cross-cultural and cross-racial encounters, the extent to which British society in general and social workers have questioned the assumptions and beliefs they hold about ethnic minorities is highly debatable, an opinion shared by Denney (1983). In a review of the literature on cross-cultural counselling, Marett identifies a continuing debate. Those such as Patterson (1978) and Sutton (1979) advocate a universalistic view of client needs, suggesting that helping relationships based on the key conditions of warmth, accurate empathy, and genuineness, and the concept of self-actualization, can be universally effective, regardless of ethnicity. Opposed to this is the special-treatment view, which suggests the need for special recognition of cultural differences and requires social workers not only to attempt to understand each culture in its own terms and the individual client's commitment to that culture, but also to examine 'all the overt and (more important) hidden assumptions of one's own cultural background' and to acknowledge how pervasively they intrude (Marett 1981:54) The universalist view is less well supported, however, and a note of caution is sounded by Marett, pointing out that there is evidence that amongst some ethnic groups, such as the Burmese, these same helping qualities might be taken as evidence of weakness and incompetence on the part of the social worker.

In the light of these issues, a more realistic approach may be the avoidance of such a dichotomy by the adoption of a view that recognizes not only the importance of an awareness of cultural differences and the impact these may have on helping relationsips and techniques, but also the importance of establishing an appropriate atmosphere in which such a relationship may flourish. This will often include warmth, genuineness, and accurate empathy, although prescriptive statements about practice are clearly problematic. Marett (1981), for example, indicates that, alongside the evidence of difficulties for white counsellors with black clients, there is also evidence that failure of a black counsellor to meet a black client's expectations may be just as traumatic. Similarly, Francis (1984a) points out that social workers from the same culture as the client may be at a *dis*advantage and be blinded by their own prejudices, and that an objective approach may be the best way to help the client to assess the cultural component of their problems.

In addition, there is also some evidence relating to the effectiveness of white counsellors with black clients suggesting that clear structuring of the client–worker relationship with an overt definition of respective roles may be one way of overcoming both cultural and psychodynamic obstacles. Marett also refers to evidence from Asian counselling encounters in British settings of expectations of concrete and well-structured situations, and a dislike of approaches that are too confrontational and emotionally intense. However, this contrasts to some extent with the experience of the NMGC Asian Project, where it has been found that many Asians seek help in crisis situations that is often short-term and crisis-related, and therefore both confrontational and intense. This results in more directive work, 'not only because of the intrinsic difficulties but also because of the expectation of parental instruction. The counsellor is seen as a substitute for the village elder' (Mitchell 1984:6). Evidence relating to practice is currently sparse and to some extent perhaps even contradictory, although not necessarily so. But it suggests that there may be a need for a clear definition of roles and expectations, and for both structure and time boundaries, which indicates that both task-centred and crisis-intervention methods may be relevant. The principles and methods of conciliation discussed in Chapter 8 may also be relevant in some marital disputes involving the extended family. This inference clearly needs substantiation, however, through both practice and research.

The use of volunteers and interpreters from local communities may also be of great value as part of a multi-faceted approach (see, for example, British Association of Social Workers 1982). Whilst no such worker can possibly meet the needs of all ethnic groups, any more than any white worker can meet the needs of all European or white communities, a worker from the community may often be in a better position to provide a helping service than someone from a totally different background, especially where there are language problems.

Lago (1981) also draws attention to fundamental communication problems such as the lack of a common language. Even the *presence* of a common language may conceal important differences in the use and understanding of common words and concepts, in the use and nature of questioning, of intonation, and of volume of speech, and even in the use and significance of certain verbal reinforcers such as grunts, all of which not only can confuse but may even cause offence to one or the other. There may also be differing patterns of non-verbal behaviour, quite apart from any confusion caused by a lack of awareness by the client of the nature of the helping process (see, for example, British Association of Social Workers 1982: appendix IV). Nevertheless, as Lago says, 'attempting to understand the client as if one were the client . . . can act as the most important single ingredient for establishing a working partnership with the client' (1981:62). For even the attempt will help to create an atmosphere of unconditional acceptance of the client and show a genuine wish to understand him, which may constitute a starting point for effective cross-cultural work.

As Cheetham (1981) and Roger Ballard (1979) suggest, it is also important to recognize and to work with the strengths of different cultural and family backgrounds. In South Asian families, for example, we have already argued that disputes almost invariably involve the extended family. Social workers may therefore have to deal with a much wider range of people than they would normally expect; but if this is taken into account and incorporated into an intervention strategy,

'then some things may go more smoothly than expected. In a world of corporate groups . . . the idea of the broker or go-between, whose task it is to find some sort of mutually acceptable compromise, is well established.' (R. Ballard 1979:154)

Faced with the complexity of the issues presented by cross-cultural social work, it is clear that there are a number of issues relating to both training and practice that need to be addressed (British Association of Social Workers 1982). A frequent response has been to call for the appointment of more specialist workers (Association of Directors of Social Services 1983). Kinnon (1984) has argued, however, that some of the assumptions underlying this reasoning are not valid, not least because of the complexity of the pattern of immigration to Britain and the many diverse cultural backgrounds to be found amongst what appear to be homogeneous ethnic minority groups. The lack of consensus makes it difficult to suggest what the most appropriate response should be, whilst lack of research makes clear statements about practice equally hard to offer. Ultimately, the relationship between client and worker remains of central importance, a relationship that will need to encompass both universal needs, and specialist needs that take full account of relevant cultural factors. At the same time, as Marett concludes:

> 'the final need must be a very clear recognition of the ever-present discrimination and prejudice faced by ethnic minority members in modern societies . . . it is of little use for counsellors and other social workers to support a client in his striving for the actualisation of his potential, without attempting to do something about the social forces that are working against him.'   (1981:57)

However, involvement in political and community action, which might be more attractive in so far as the issues and obstacles often seem more readily identifiable, but which fails to recognize the need for and value of individual help, would be equally one-sided.

8
Conciliation

Our major focus so far has been upon intervention in marital problems with a view to helping to resolve, or at least ease, them. Relationships sometimes deteriorate to such an extent, however, that their dissolution becomes inevitable. There is therefore an argument for some intervention to be directed towards minimizing the disruptive consequences of marital and family breakdown, a view held by the Finer Committee (DHSS 1974), since this represents, both literally and figuratively, the ultimate problem faced by any marriage. Conciliation differs fundamentally from other approaches that have been discussed because, apart from intrinsic differences, it is a developing area of practice, emerging from dissatisfaction with the present legal system and a search for an alternative, rather than from an established area of social work practice or an established body of social work theory.

The attempt to achieve settlement of disputes through negotiation rather than conflict is not a new concept in the field of either interpersonal relationships or industrial/economic relationships (Gulliver 1979). Nor indeed is it entirely new in relation to divorce, having existed in parts of the United States since 1939 (Forster 1982), although in most modern industrialized areas of the world the major expansion of such practices has occurred since 1970. In Britain, development has been somewhat slower, because until 1970 collusion was a bar to divorce. The concept was first mooted by the Finer Committee, but its first real application came with the formation of the Bristol Courts Family Conciliation Service in 1978, in response to these proposals. Since these are the starting point, it is worth noting their definition of conciliation as a process of

'assisting the parties to deal with the consequences of the established breakdown of their marriage, whether resulting in a divorce
or separation, by reaching agreements or giving consents or reducing
the area of conflict upon custody, support, access to and education of
the children, financial provision, the disposition of the matrimonial
home, lawyers' fees, and every other matter arising from the breakdown which calls for a decision on future arrangements'.

(DHSS1974:176)

It is interesting that, more than ten years later, the Booth Committee
has chosen to adopt the same definition in its discussion of conciliation (Lord Chancellor's Department 1985: para. 3.10).

It has been argued (Roberts 1983) that, whilst the concept underlying this definition of conciliation – i.e. the desirability of families,
rather than judges, reaching decisions about their own future – is
simple and attractive, the definition is less than helpful, since it does
not suggest how this might be effected. In consequence,

'it is difficult to isolate a consistent package of ideas associated with
this movement . . . when the embryonic institutions of "conciliation"
now beginning to operate are examined, considerable diversity is
also observable . . . from general counselling and advice to detailed
work on specific issues; and approaches appear to differ from unob-
trusive aids to communication to pressure-laden directive intervention.'

(Roberts 1983:537 – 38)

As a result, it is possible to identify at least four different approaches to
conciliation in Britain: a growing number of independent 'out-of-
court' conciliation services (mostly voluntary and offering free or below-
cost services) usually operating before court proceedings are fully under
way, of which there are currently some twenty-four in existence (Parkinson 1986a); conciliation by probation officers whilst preparing welfare reports, a widespread and widely supported practice (James and
Wilson 1984a); conciliation by probation officers specializing in
divorce-court welfare work, perhaps through specialist civil work
teams, as part of an 'in-court' conciliation process in the sense that it
arises out of a court-orientated process; and conciliation by judges,
registrars, and/or divorce-court welfare officers, which are 'in-court'
schemes, operating on and from court premises as part of the divorce
process in those courts, as with the Bristol courts and the scheme operated by the Principal Registry of the Family Division of the High Court.

Such a wide range of approaches leads to much conceptual and
semantic confusion. This, apart from its impace on the development

of practice, makes debate about the subject difficult and potentially misleading. It is essential therefore to broach some of these issues before beginning to explore the contribution and place of social work in conciliation.

Conciliation: concepts, context, and clarification

The first distinction to be drawn is between reconciliation and conciliation, since the two are frequently confused. Reconciliation refers primarily to reuniting spouses facing marital conflict and potential dissolution of their relationship, whilst conciliation is concerned with helping couples to separate with as little conflict as possible. Further distinctions should also be made, in order to clarify the current debate about conciliation, since the term is used to describe an *objective*, a *process*, and a *method*. Thus, the growth of divorce counselling, which may occur after the marriage and the family have split up, may be described as conciliation in so far as its objective is reducing both interpersonal and intrapersonal conflict, with the aim of easing the emotional impact of divorce and any resulting conflict. Parkinson (1985b) discusses such developments in some detail, and the approaches described in earlier chapters may also be relevant. Similarly, the work undertaken by many probation officers whilst preparing welfare reports, which some solicitors also attempt, involving encouraging each spouse to recognize and respect the other's position by acting as an intermediary in the hope of reducing conflict, may be described as conciliation in the sense that it is part of a *process* of being conciliatory. Conciliation is also used to describe a *method* of working, in which a conciliator uses a particular approach as part of an explicit process of dispute management and conflict resolution. It is with conciliation in this sense that we are primarily concerned in this chapter.

The system of family law in Britain is rooted in an adversarial model of justice. This is founded on the assumption that, where a dispute exists, the fairest and most just outcome is achieved through a contest between the parties, the result of which will be determined by someone sitting in judgement. In spite of recent changes, the 1969 Divorce Reform Act perpetuates *in reality* the principle of the matrimonial offence, thereby stimulating conflict from the start of proceedings. As Davis has commented, 'The legal framework as a whole may appear clumsy and inappropriate as a means of settling issues which have such a high emotional content' (1983:6), not least because, as he has pointed out elsewhere, 'The procedure is not designed to cater for the family as a whole' (Davis 1982b:356); it focusses primarily on the dissolution of the marriage rather than on the splitting up of the family.

Whilst conciliation has not been accepted without criticism (e.g. Bottomley 1984, Roberts 1983), and Freeman has argued against 'rampant interventionism' and that 'the family, particularly its weaker members, will suffer further from delegalisation' (1984:19), the adversarial approach of the legal system appears ill-suited to the many situations in divorce where a clean break is not possible and the desirability of continuing post-divorce relationships between parents and children (and therefore parent and parent) is recognized. Furthermore, the main issues in many divorces revolve around the children: 'In these circumstances, procedures designed to unravel complicated family fortunes can seem wasteful and irrelevant' (Davis 1982b: 6), because the dispute is much more likely to reflect emotional responses than economic facts. Moreover, as Parkinson has argued,

> 'an adversarial legal process can unleash destructive impulses of frightening intensity. . . . Although children's welfare is paramount in law . . . in the intensity of marital strife, little attention may be paid to the children's needs.'   (1983a:19—20)

Thus an adversarial process can be more than simply inappropriate; it can be counter-productive in terms of settling a dispute and protecting children's interests. Its impact on family decisions is marginal, since Eekelaar and Clive (1977) have shown that courts often ratify the arrangements already made by the parents, thereby preserving the status quo. Therefore, as we have argued elsewhere (James and Wilson 1984c, 1984d), decisions made early in the process of separation, especially those concerning custody and access, are crucial in terms of determining the eventual outcome of many court hearings, rather than vice versa. This underlines the fact that

> 'the family itself represents a private ordering system that has the capacity of resolving its own disputes . . . and the state has a strong interest in supporting the family as an indigenous dispute resolution mechanism.'   (Sander 1984: xii)

Some further distinctions may usefully be drawn between various methods of dispute settlement, since this is yet another area where conceptual and semantic confusion abounds. The definitions we draw and the distinctions we seek to make, although partially echoed by others (Parkinson 1985a, Roberts 1983, Sander 1984), are far from being universally accepted, but the undiscriminating use of a number of different terms suggests that part of the confusion and uncertainty in practice stems from a lack of conceptual clarity. The effort to draw distinctions may therefore be worthwhile.

NEGOTIATION

Negotiation is a term best used to describe the parties' own attempts to settle their dispute. Lawyers may be involved in negotiations, representing their respective clients' interests, but such negotiations are usually a formal prelude to a contest and as such 'are an inadequate substitute for discussion between husband and wife' (Parkinson 1983a: 20). Whilst direct negotiations between spouses are desirable, since consensual agreements are clearly preferable, it is nevertheless apparent that inequalities in bargaining power between the parties do exist: e.g. unequal control over or access to financial resources; *de facto* custody of the children; emotional or intellectual dominance; and, as Parkinson (1983b) has pointed out, actual or threatened violence. Decisions negotiated early in the process of marital breakdown will therefore often reflect the interplay of these various factors, since a key feature of negotiation is the absence of the involvement of a third party, and the process is controlled entirely by the parties or by their lawyers, which Roberts (1983) refers to as 'supported negotiations'.

CONCILIATION

Conciliation is crucially different from negotiation because of the intervention of a neutral third party whose role is to help the couple towards an agreed outcome. The conciliator is not a unilateral decision-maker but a facilitator

'of the process leading to the parties' joint decision. In various ways they help to increase or orient the exchange of information and to expedite the learning and adjustment process. Their presence does not deprive the disputants of the final ability, or need, to make their own individual choices and to reach an agreed decision.'

(Gulliver 1979:6)

The main elements of this method involve helping the couple to communicate and to clarify facts, feelings, interactions, options, and objectives, together with a consideration of the legal issues and their implications with the aim, through participative decision-making, of assisting the family to reorganize. A third party affects not only the interpersonal dynamics but also the procedural nature of the decision-making process. Thus, procedural agreements will be negotiated with the parties, which are important, not only in terms of agreeing a framework for the discussions, but because 'each joint decision . . . contributes to the development of a coordination between them that is essential to the ultimate end of an agreed outcome' (Gulliver 1979:7).

MEDIATION

Much of what has been said above of conciliation can also be said of mediation, and indeed some authors (e.g. Davis 1983, Folberg and Taylor 1984) imply a degree of interchangeability between the two terms. It is however between these terms in particular that the greatest confusion exists. Thus Folberg and Taylor describe mediation as a method to 'maximise the exploration of alternatives' (1984:9), whilst Haynes describes a process of mediation that may require the mediator at times to 'lean on one party to move from an unreasonable position' or to suggest 'strategies to the other party that increase that party's power in relation to the spouse' (1981:127). It is unclear whether these two approaches to mediation are seen to be compatible, but the Haynes approach describes a style of intervention corresponding to Roberts's 'pressure laden directive intervention', which we would argue is not conciliation. In contrast, Coogler (1978) advocates a highly structured approach to mediation and regards conciliation as different in offering options for the parties to consider, pointing out the advantages and disadvantages of various alternatives, and maybe encouraging the parties to adopt an available option rather than remain at an impasse. He concludes that conciliation takes over 'the parties' responsibility for examining the issues and discovering options. Conciliation is thus a less desirable option than mediation and serves as an alternative to an impasse' (Coogler 1978:3). Haynes's notion of 'leaning' on parties in mediation, on the other hand, seems a more intrusive means of resolving an impasse than suggesting options and exploring their relative advantages and disadvantages.

There appears to be no consensus about appropriate distinctions, then, although we believe that two important points can be made. First, Coogler, Folberg, and Taylor, and Haynes all describe mediation as a process in which the degree of structure imposed in the proceedings is substantially greater than in much of the conciliation practised in Britain. We would consequently suggest that mediation might be represented as a more structured and more formalized approach. Second, it has been suggested (Davis and Bader, 1983) that the term 'mediation' might be more appropriately used in Britain in relation to in-court schemes, especially those operating from court premises with court officials such as registrars and welfare officers. These may be seen as more formal and more structured, since, as Gulliver has stated, 'The locus of decision making, together with the process leading to it and affected by it, is taken to be crucial' (1979:3). It is interesting that mediation in the United States is often more clearly orientated towards the legal process by seeking agreement on *all* contested issues, including financial and property matters which are commonly not dealt with by conciliation in Britain. We would suggest therefore that whilst conciliation has some structure, this is less formal, less predetermined, and more open to negotiation than mediation, and that although the two terms have been seen as synonymous, greater clarity would result from a consistent differentiation between the concepts such as that suggested.

ARBITRATION

The distinctive feature of arbitration is that, whilst the arbitrator may facilitate a process whereby disputants are encouraged to settle their differences, ultimately he has the power to make a decision that will bind the parties. Such proceedings are likely to be more formal, in the sense that the arbitrator is vested with substantial authority and is likely to be perceived by the parties as representing the formal process. Also, the parties may be accompanied by legal or other representatives, since the proceedings may have strong judicial overtones, even though they may not be conducted in the formal setting of a court of law.

ADJUDICATION

This is the method that currently exists for settling disputes. It is both structured and formal, involving a hearing at which a decision is imposed by a judicial third party in order to settle the dispute. It is also the method in which the parties have the least control over either the procedures or the outcome.

In the light of this analysis, we would argue that these various methods can be placed along a continuum derived from certain key characteristics, such as the degree of formality. Although, as Roberts (1983) argues, adjudicatory proceedings with a high level of informality can be devised, formality is also a function of the parties' perceptions of the nature and extent of the authority present. This in turn is related to the role and authority of the conciliator in comparison with that of an arbitrator or adjudicator, who has the authority to make a decision. Similarly, differences in the structure of proceedings and the degree of control over this are also reflections of formality, from the least structured process of negotiation, through conciliation and mediation where the couple control the proceedings to varying degrees, to adjudication where the structure is highly formalized and almost totally imposed on the parties. The final important characteristic is the degree of voluntarism, in the sense that negotiation and conciliation are almost entirely voluntary, but the closer dispute settlement methods are to the formal legal system, the greater the degree of compulsion may seem to become.

Thus at one end of the continuum lies negotiation, which is voluntary and informal, where the proceedings are controlled by the parties, and the authority for any decision is derived from their mutual consent. At the other end lies adjudication, which is compulsory and highly formal, in which the structure of the proceedings is imposed totally from without and is defined in great detail, and where the authority to enforce any decision lies, in principle, in the entire system of common and statute law that underpins our legal system. In between lie the other approaches, in which, to varying degrees, there is 'bargaining in the shadow of the law' (Mnookin and Kornhauser 1979). Conciliation lies, we would argue, towards the lower end of this continuum, where 'the shadow of the law' is not so deep. Certainly, all agreements must be sanctioned and ratified by the courts, since divorce is a legal as well as an emotional process and there are clear issues and principles of justice involved: 'Conciliation is an alternative to contested court proceedings, not a substitute for legal advice and assistance' (Parkinson 1983a: 23). Moreover, whilst property issues may be few in most divorces, and conciliation may well establish an atmosphere in which even these issues can be settled, it may be that in some cases such matters are more appropriately dealt with through a more formal and structured process. Conciliation, however, encourages the parties to participate in the process by working towards objectives that they help to define, through procedures that they agree, with the aim of reaching their own decision.

Roberts (1983) has suggested that some of the benefits proposed for a move towards 'private ordering' through conciliation are partly illusory, in that the admission of the failure of negotiation and the decision to involve a third party result in not only some *loss* of control over the proceedings, but also an alteration of the distribution of power. Negotiation often fails precisely because of an imbalance of power, however, and the presence of a conciliator can provide a regulating function without resorting to law. Any reduction of control over this process is the result of a voluntary acceptance of this by both parties, rather than the almost total loss of control that is an inevitable consequence of an adjudicatory process. He also argues that 'Insofar as the mediator succeeds in transforming the disputants' views of the quarrel, he comes to share with them control over the outcome' (Roberts 1983: 549). If the role of the conciliator is to facilitate the couple's efforts to reach an agreement, however, control will be limited to the process, whilst the *nature* and *content* of that agreement remain entirely within the control of the parties.

Principles of conciliation

It is apparent from an overview of these issues that the argument for the move towards private ordering of family disputes, although given added impetus by dissatisfaction with the inability of the present system to cope adequately and sensitively with the issues raised, is not derived solely from such influences. It is also strongly influenced by the emergence from the debate of positive principles that take into account the continuity of biological ties within family relationships and therefore the need to seek settlements with a high level of mutual agreement and commitment, through a process containing or even reducing conflict, rather than exacerbating it. Such principles are in evidence in the recent proposals of the Booth Committee (Lord Chancellor's Department 1985: part III) for a fresh approach to the law relating to marital breakdown.

The first such principle is that parenting is the responsibility of both parents and that it is therefore their responsibility to reach decisions about custody and access arrangements for their children. This reflects the view that parenting continues even when the spousal relationship ends, and that divorce is not about loss but reorganization, both of parental responsibilities and family life. As Ahrons (1980) has suggested, what may emerge is a reorganized 'binuclear family', where one family is split between two households and in which both parents continue to have important roles in relation to their children.

The second principle is that parents should be encouraged and supported in their attempts to shoulder this responsibility and that it is inappropriate for any third party to assume this responsibility until every alternative has been explored. Whilst children are intimately involved, it is inappropriate for this burden to be placed upon their shoulders, or to be given to the courts. It is, however, a heavy responsibility, in which parents can be supported.

The third principle is that post-separation parenting should be as positive as possible if the best interests of the children are to be provided for. Various studies (James and Wilson 1984c, Richards and Dyson 1982, Rutter 1975, Walczak with Burns 1984, Wallerstein and Kelly 1980) have drawn attention to the negative impact that parental conflict – in addition to the disruption that inevitably follows separation and divorce – can have upon children.

The fourth principle is that the primary purpose of conciliation is to reach agreements, in order to help families to reorganize with the minimum amount of damage to their members. Whilst there may be continuing underlying conflicts about the breakdown of the marital relationship, these are relevant only in so far as they are obstacles to an agreement. Disagreements, particularly over children, often reflect underlying conflicts or an unwillingness to let go of the marital relationship. If these are left unacknowledged, agreement may be hard to reach or superficial and short-lived; none the less, conciliation is essentially concerned with reaching agreements rather than providing therapy. Since this distinction raises important issues, we will return to it in more detail later.

The fifth principle, derived from the others, is that conciliation is a more effective way of achieving the other principles than an adversarial approach, and that since conciliation should assist families in resolving their disputes, all members of the nuclear family should be involved in the process in order to foster interaction and co-operation, and that members of the extended family should also be involved if necessary in order to facilitate the process of reaching an agreement. This point will also be returned to in more detail later.

The theoretical bases of conciliation and their implications for practice

It is important to restate that conciliation has its roots in a changing view of the legal response to marital breakdown and not in an existing area of social work practice or theory. There is therefore no social work theory intrinsic to conciliation, a fact that underlies much of the diversity of practice. Indeed, as Davis (1983) has argued, it is misleading to think of conciliation as the sole preserve of the social work profession, even though many conciliators are social workers, since it can also involve both lawyers and legal administrators, who also have strong claims to a legitimate involvement in conciliation. We are primarily concerned here, however, with the contribution of social work and the identification of social work theory and knowledge that might be appropriately related to conciliation, not only as a source of clarification but also as a potential source of enrichment for the structuring and practice of conciliation.

CRISIS INTERVENTION

A detailed discussion of the theory of crisis intervention can be found in Chapter 6. Its relevance to conciliation is substantial. Crisis theory assumes, for example, that part of the psychological response to the challenge of a crisis is one of increased problem-solving activity during the early stages of the response to the crisis. This can be harnessed in conciliation. In addition, in view of the concept of marital breakdown as a crisis matrix consisting of a series of recurring short-lived crises, the implication – bearing in mind the resurrection of previously learned coping mechanisms during a crisis – is that any helping process is likely to be more effective if healthy adaptive coping mechanisms are encouraged at an early point in the crisis matrix. As Parkinson has argued, therefore,

'Conciliation should be available to the parties at an early stage . . . and should be quickly accessible in crisis situations. . . . The stage at which conciliation is begun is an important factor in its outcome.'
(1983a:24)

Whilst the validity of this last assertion remains to be empirically demonstrated, when this perspective is juxtaposed with the argument outlined above concerning the importance of decisions made early in the process of separation and the difficulty of subsequently reversing such decisions, a powerful argument emerges for conciliation early on in the divorce process. This view is shared by the Booth Committee (Lord Chancellor's Department 1985: para. 3.12).

TASK-CENTRED INTERVENTION

The theory of task-centred intervention, which is discussed in more detail in Chapter 6, also has much of relevance to offer conciliation. Kelly has argued that conciliation is 'a goal-focussed, task-oriented, time limited process. It emphasises the present and the future, not the past. Crisis and short-term therapy share some of these parameters' (1983:35). Parkinson (1983a) and Folberg and Taylor (1984) agree with this view. The notion of brief, time-limited intervention is thus an important one in relation to conciliation, suggesting major assumptions about practice – e.g. that it is the client who defines the problem and has the capacity to respond to the challenge and resolve it, with the facilitation of the conciliator; and that conciliation does not require investigation and enquiry into past events, except in so far as they are relevant to the present problem, nor any attempt to 'diagnose' the problem, whilst the client remains the main 'change agent'.

Task-centred work is considered especially appropriate for intervention with a range of problems, many of which may arise in marital breakdown and some of which occur frequently in conciliation. It also relies more heavily on techniques aimed at encouraging a cognitive grasp of reality which, as we have argued, is important during the crisis of marital breakdown, rather than techniques for increasing the client's self-awareness as an end in itself. In conciliation, however, these constraints must be applied to the family and not just to individual clients, a transposition that alters the dynamic nature of the process.

PROBLEM-SOLVING

Conciliation has already been referred to as a process of problem-solving. Perlman's (1957) theory, which focusses upon the client's problem-solving ability and asserts that problems in living can only be resolved, occasionally with outside assistance, by those who experience them, and which also accepts the client's definition of the problem as the main focus, is thus also relevant. It also stresses the importance of a warm, empathetic, and genuinely caring relationship in the helping process, as well as the view that people are constantly in the process of becoming and growing, with the result that even partial solutions that ease problems are of value. Perlman also emphasizes the need to make the problem to be worked upon as explicit and clearly defined as possible in relation to what can realistically be done about it, without the need for an extensive 'diagnostic' phase at the beginning of the process. In this sense, it recognizes the need to respond to the whole person, whilst at the same time acknowledging the value of partializing problematic experiences. It also highlights the need to recognize 'the place' as an important variable in the helping process, in the sense that the agency setting exerts important but diffuse organizational pressures on the helping process, which may be to do with structure or resources. The significance of this looms large when we consider conciliation as it is developing in the probation service and also in some in-court schemes.

FAMILY THERAPY

Parkinson has also drawn attention to the importance of perspectives derived from family therapy to the practice of conciliation, since it is essentially conjoint work with both partners.

> 'The nature of the family interaction and of underlying pathology should be recognized, if possible, because an understanding of their influence may be essential to effective conciliation, although *it is not the direct focus of the work.*'
>
> (Parkinson 1983a:25, emphasis added)

Since conciliation is concerned with family break-up and reorganization, an approach that encourages the family to be conceived of as a system to be viewed as a whole is clearly of relevance, particularly in terms of shedding light on the dynamic nature of family interactions and the uniqueness of family communication patterns.

Two other points also emerge, both of which we will consider in more detail later. The first is the importance of distinguishing between perspectives and techniques derived from family therapy that can be applied in conciliation, and the use of family therapy as a form of treatment. To suggest that

> 'the marital relationship system heavily influences the management of individual and family development tasks and that to understand the problems of the individual and the family it is necessary to understand the nature of the marriage'   (Scherz 1970:226)

is an argument that valuable insights might be obtained from family therapy, but not that conciliation should involve the practice of family therapy. The second point is that this perspective highlights the importance of working not just with the marital dyad, but with the children and other members of the immediate family system. Perspectives derived from family therapy will be of little value if children are not involved, although the nature and extent of their involvement must be carefully considered.

BEHAVIOURAL APPROACHES

Although the impact of behavioural thinking on conciliation is seldom explicit, there are elements (see Chapter 3) that are relevant in understanding and developing methods of conciliation. Conciliation is focussed very much on present events and responses, rather than on the past. Many of the techniques are therefore aimed at influencing the contemporary sustaining conditions in which various negative behaviours occur, often focussing upon observable responses and behaviour and on attempts to modify these by using verbal reinforcers for positive responses and not reinforcing negative responses in order to minimize or extinguish the latter. Conciliation also sets clear behavioural goals in terms of achieving positive approaches to post-divorce parenting, new behavioural responses, and reaching clearly stated agreements, and might involve techniques such as agreeing short-term goals or tasks to be worked upon between sessions as part of the process of building up confidence and trust whilst working towards an eventual agreement. Inter-spousal behaviour during the process of marital breakdown may therefore become an important focus for the intervention of conciliators; a full and useful discussion of the kind of behaviour and strategies often used by partners in an attempt to influence the process is offered by Saposnek (1983).

Arising both from these theoretical perspectives and from the nature and demands of conciliation are a number of attributes and techniques of particular relevance and importance to such work. Amongst the most crucial of these is the neutrality of the conciliator, an attribute on which all commentators are agreed and upon which the Booth Committee comments (Lord Chancellor's Department 1985: para. 3.10), although it is not unproblematic (see Bernard et al. 1984). Haynes (1981) has argued that rather than aiming for neutrality, which is very difficult to achieve and sustain, the conciliator should maintain a careful balance between the couple and try to be even-handed in giving support, encouragement, and praise, and to be seen as non-partisan and committed to reaching an agreement rather than to either party. The use of co-workers may be important to this end, since a co-worker can identify and respond to any apparent lack of even-handedness, an approach recommended by Waldron et al. (1984), Guise (1983), and others. The presence of a co-worker is also of great value in terms of keeping track of the processes of interaction and as a partial safeguard against becoming enmeshed in the family's problems and struggles, whilst the opportunity to reflect with a co-worker upon progress, or lack of it, is a valuable source of insight and support. A practice that many co-workers find helpful as a means of achieving this is to take some time out together during the session, having explained at the outset that this might occur. Particularly in the early stages of a co-working partnership, it may be easiest to do this as a matter of routine before a final agreement is reached to ensure that both feel that there are no outstanding issues.

Another key issue in conciliation, given the emotional state of people in crisis and the threat and fear of losing control, is the management of conflict: maintaining firm but flexible control over the proceedings and ensuring that the couple know that this will be sustained; making judgements about the amount of anger and sadness that may need to be expressed before one or both are ready to listen to each other, and about the point at which the conciliators need to intervene; and so on. Parkinson, underlining the importance of clarification in the process, argues that 'Conflict often results from failed communication rather than from incompatible values and goals. Conciliation helps to reveal mistaken assumptions and perceptions' (1983a:32). Haynes (1983) also stresses the importance of the parties having as much information as possible about each other's feelings and positions, in order that these might be clarified so that *unnecessary* conflict might be avoided. This raises an important issue, since

> 'where there has been marital breakdown, it is "necessary" for the parties to get the anger and sadness off their chests . . . before it is possible for them to set about agreeing upon continuing aspects of their relationship.'   (Roberts 1983:539)

Conciliators must be able to cope with their own feelings about conflict and the need to control it, in order that this necessary conflict can be allowed and even facilitated, without it turning into destructive conflict such as that produced by an adversarial approach.

Kelly (1983) suggests several other strategies for conflict management. The importance of a win–win philosophy should be stressed, in which neither the parents nor the children are the losers and in which mutual needs are met. She also argues that particular techniques can be helpful, such as asking a parent to justify the demands they are making, or to explain why the other parent should accept a particular proposal. This is important in terms of helping each parent to see the situation from the other's point of view, and is a safeguard for the conciliators against trying to persuade the parents to 'see sense' (or to see it from the conciliators' point of view), as opposed to making the some-times considerable effort to see the situation from their point of view. It also serves to reinforce the conciliators' neutrality. Other techniques may help to pre-empt unnecessary conflict, which is preferable to trying to control it once it has escalated. The conciliators may anticipate and state a parent's thoughts, feelings, or responses in order to neutralize an adverse reaction before it occurs. Making such feelings an explicit focus for discussion, when they seem likely to block progress if they are not acknowledged, also helps the conciliators to keep the initiative and maintain control.

Similarly, giving information such as the importance to children of continued positive contact with *both* parents can pre-empt or make more difficult any move by the parent with *de facto* custody to argue that the children do not need the other parent. Information can also be given about options such as joint custody orders, where both parents have custody whilst one retains care and control. Use of terminology in such situations is also an issue of sensitivity. Patrician has concluded that

'there are significant differences in connotation between the terms *joint legal custody* and *sole legal custody* and between the terms *custodial parent* and *non-custodial parent*.'   (1984:55)

The symbolic importance of joint custody and the use of terms such as 'parent', instead of 'party', should therefore not be overlooked. Infor-mation about what is going to happen, what reactions might be expected from the children, and even what others in similar situations have experienced and how they have resolved their problems might also usefully be given.

In handling conflict, it is important to maintain a focus on the pre-sent and the future. 'As a rule, couples are not encouraged to explore past differences unless it helps them to resolve current issues' (Blades 1984:83). Any other work with such problems should be separated from conciliation and dealt with by more appropriate methods on other occasions, by other workers, or even by other agencies. Focuss-ing on the past tends to heighten conflict, to lead to accusations, and to stress differences, whilst the conciliators should be striving to focus upon similarities, upon strengths, and upon what is agreed. Allied to this is the need to offer positive reinforcement to constructive atti-tudes that might facilitate agreement by complimenting, praising, and underlining strengths. This is important, not only because it helps to reduce conflict, since it is difficult to sustain anger and be defensive whilst being praised, but it also improves self-esteem and the sense of coping, which can be severely undermined during the process of marital breakdown. Positive parenting attributes and attitudes of *both* parents are major targets for such reinforcement, provided this is given genuinely and in moderation.

The technique of reframing, which was discussed in Chapter 5, is also helpful in keeping the atmosphere positive and constructive and in maintaining the focus on the children's needs. Thus, the question/assertion 'Why can you never collect the children on time? You're always late!' can be intercepted by the conciliators, who might respond by asking, 'Are you suggesting that the children would be happier if they weren't kept waiting and uncertain about whether they will be picked up?' Similarly, the common assertion that 'The children are always upset when they leave me!' – which is usually countered by a similar statement by the other parent – can be reframed by suggesting, 'It is obvious that the children love you both and want to be with you both.'

General skills, such as the use of questions, may also be used in a specific way to direct and control the interaction, since questions not only elicit information but make statements about what information is important to the questioner. Closed questions, seeking factual information, may help to control a repetitive or counter-productive focus on emotions. When a parent complains, 'Why can you never bring the children back at the agreed time?' the question 'How does that make you feel?' will produce a very different response from the question 'What time would you like them to be brought back and how flexible can this be?' The latter focusses not upon feelings of frustration and conflict, but upon facts and the need to generate agreement by helping the parents to formulate their own solutions. Similarly, aggressive or hurtful comments such as the accusation that 'You never spent any time with the children before, so why the great interest now?' can be extremely counter-productive and may need to be deflected by an interjection such as 'It's natural to feel hurt and angry right now, but often a parent will feel differently after a separation. Making it possible for the children to spend time with them now might make up for what you feel they have missed in the past, and may be especially important to them in the present circumstances.'

Other skills, such as addressing comments to both parents, respectful attending, paraphrasing, reflection of feeling, and sustaining procedures, are invaluable. The channels of communication can also be controlled so that, as Blades suggests, when discussions are going smoothly husband and wife can communicate directly with one another, with the conciliators helping them to 'clarify agreements, redirect the conversation when they lose sight of their task, and cut short arguments when they are not productive' (1984:75). If conflict begins to escalate, however, the conciliators may seek a more structured approach so that couples may be asked to address comments through conciliators, to speak only one at a time and refrain from interrupting, or refrain from referring to past events and problems – in other words, to agree to any rules that might control unnecessary conflict and facilitate the process of working towards an agreement (see also Coogler 1978). In addition, the non-verbal aspects of interaction should be fully used to facilitate the process and to control conflict, even to the extent of altering the seating arrangements, standing physically between two embattled parents, or leaving the room, although recourse to such extreme measures should not be needed often. If the process really does become stuck, it may be helpful to offer carefully balanced suggestions, to explore a range of different time-sharing methods, to refer to solutions reached by other parents, and to reiterate the importance of mutually agreed decisions for the welfare of the children.

Such techniques, although not unique to conciliation, imply that the conciliator may need to be much more active in controlling the process than is common in much social work practice. Roberts argues that the extent to which conciliators 'should seek to regulate the inter-action between the disputants and to assert control over the outcome' (1983:551) is a question that needs to be faced, but this is to confuse two separate issues: control over the *process*, which is appropriate, as opposed to control over the *outcome*, which is not, since this must be determined by the parents. Saposnek regards the effective conciliator as being active, assertive, goal-orientated, and business-like in order to

'deal with the emotional aspects of the process without allowing them to disrupt the problem-solving. Too tight control restricts the complexity of the emotional issues . . . while too loose control allows the emotional charge to overwhelm the rational structure needed to reach resolution.'   (1983:32)

From the principles and processes outlined above, it is apparent that conciliation is not a process of therapy and that to work 'at greater lengths with . . . [some families] on a therapeutic basis by using the family therapy approach' (Guise 1983:59) is to confuse the two in a way that exposes conciliation to unnecessary criticism of uncertainty about its methods and objectives. This distinction is made in the pro-posals of the Booth Committee (Lord Chancellor's Department 1985:

para 3.11), whilst Rosanova has also argued that conciliation is not therapy, and that, whilst understanding therapeutic techniques may be advantageous, the conciliator has 'no right to find individual behaviour healthy or pathological, or to convince clients to amend general patterns of behaviour, or to undertake searches for unconscious motives' (1983:64). Indeed, to attempt therapeutic intervention when conciliation is expected may even be counter-productive.

Similarly, whilst Kelly emphasizes the need to make continuous and impartial judgements about how much emotional expression and exploration is really needed in order to facilitate reaching an agreement, she concludes that conciliation is about 'helping clients to resolve their disputes and reach an acceptable agreement . . . and within that context to allow the process to be psychologically beneficial as well' (1983:37−8). This highlights the important distinction that, whilst the primary objective and the techniques and skills of conciliation are explicitly concerned with reaching agreements, it may implicitly contribute to a helping process. This view is succinctly expressed by Sander, arguing that although it 'is not therapy, it certainly can be a therapeutic experience. It can also be an important learning experience' (1984:xiii).

Another contentious issue, to which we referred earlier, concerns the nature and extent of the involvement of children in conciliation. Guise (1983) and Howard and Shepherd (1982) believe that it is important to involve children from the outset: 'Normally children are well aware of the parental conflict and can make valuable contributions, either verbally or, more often, non-verbally' (Howard and Shepherd 1982:88). Thus a mother who is resisting or making difficult access by the father, rationalizing this by arguing that the child does not want it or becomes upset by it, may find it hard to deny the significance of the child going to sit on father's knee, or snuggling up next to him. To expose children to what may be a painful process for parents might seem harmful, but it is doubtful whether they will see anything they have not seen before, with the possible exception of their parents striving to agree, without fighting, which they may well not have seen for some time. As Guise says, 'it is essential to have the children present; in their absence, there is a hazard of them becoming merely prizes to be bargained for and won or lost' (1983:58).

The involvement of children in conciliation helps to avoid this, by providing a powerful physical presence to underline the principles of parental responsibility for decision-making, the need for positive post-divorce parenting, and family reorganization rather than marital dissolution. Although there is general support for the necessity of involving the children at some point in the process, however, there is a divergence of opinion as to the extent and timing of this involvement. Coogler, for example, argues that 'parents should be encouraged to bring the children to all . . . sessions regarding custody and visitation, if they are old enough to comprehend what is happening' (1978:21). Waldron *et al.* (1984) advocate that all of the children should be seen with the parents part of the time (and sometimes alone). Walczak and Burns also suggest: 'It is a good assumption that no child is ever too young to be spoken to even if it cannot grasp all that is said' (1984:124–25).

If, as we have argued, it is the right of children to be present, this must be underlined from the outset by practice that assumes their presence to be the norm. Divergence from this should occur only when the situation seems to demand it (e.g. where there are 'couple' issues concerning the disintegration of the husband–wife relationship, which must be resolved before agreement seeking can begin, and where there may be particularly bitter conflict).

We have referred elsewhere (James and Wilson 1984c) to the involvement of children by their parents in decisions over custody and especially access. Our findings have tended to support the conclusion of Walczak and Burns (1984) that good and open communication within the family at the time of separation can help children to cope with the disruption in their lives. Their study revealed that, whilst children did not want to know in great detail why their parents were separating, many of them did

> 'like to be involved in arrangements for custody and access. . . . They want to know that the parents agree about the arrangements whatever their current relationship. . . . It is to parents that children look for explanation of things they do not understand . . . . These questions may never be asked without strong encouragement . . . that it is all right to ask and that the parent will not be angry.'
>   (Walczak and Burns 1984:59–60)

Conciliation can provide the forum and the means whereby this can occur. Walczak and Burns conclude that many more children would have been helped and would have been less confused, lonely, angry, and damaged had their parents also received help.

A distinction needs to be drawn, however, between the children's involvement in the process of conciliation and their involvement in the actual decision-making. Whilst, as Walczak and Burns argue, 'Children's wishes need *to be taken into account* when considering the future' (1984:124–25, emphasis added), the final decisions about future arrangements must be made by the parents. Handing the responsibility for crucial decisions concerning custody and access to the children is contrary to the first principle of conciliation and would be an abrogation of parental responsibilities, as well as placing children in the impossible position of having to choose between parents. Such behaviour may also enable a parent who is opposed to access to disguise this by placing the responsibility for the refusal on the children, a strategy frequently encountered by conciliators where access arrangements have broken down. It is important in such situations to point out to parents that the ultimate responsibility for the continuation of access lies with them, although genuine cases of child refusal present different problems.

The need to involve children receives theoretical support from family systems theory, in so far as this recognizes that a child can often be 'an *innocent but functional contributor* to conflict between the parents' (Saposnek 1983:120, emphasis in original). Given the confusion and upset often surrounding children in such situations, it is important to acknowledge that, in attempting to have their needs met, children may initiate and perpetuate behaviour that leads to parental conflict or exacerbates existing conflicts. Statements from children about where they want to live, for example, may well have such an effect on parents, who may need help from the conciliators to understand the motives that might underlie such behaviour, such as the common desire amongst children of all ages to see their parents reunited. Saposnek discusses a variety of strategies that children might use as part of their struggle to cope, concluding, 'Because the child's problems are embedded in the family's dynamics, it is important that those problems be viewed within the context of the family system' (1983:134).

Evidence concerning the effectiveness of conciliation, especially in Britain, is scarce. In the United States, Waldron *et al.* (1984) reported positive responses from parents and children where agreement had been reached. Folberg and Taylor (1984) reported that preliminary studies on the effect of mediation schemes in Atlanta, Denver, Maine, Portland, and Toronto, amongst others, all show a high rate of success in achieving settlements, although the rates do vary, concluding that it is an effective method of dispute settlement. Pearson and Thoennes comment that 'Despite its growing popularity and use, there have been few studies to empirically assess mediation' (1984:500), but they conclude from their study that 'Successful mediation clients maintain a number of very desirable behaviours and attitudes over time'

(1984:510). Such clients were more optimistic about being able to resolve any future difficulties, more satisfied with court orders confirming the agreed settlement, and least likely to report difficulties. They were also more likely to report a high level of compliance with orders and to enjoy good relationships with ex-partners, resulting in more contact with the children and less subsequent use of court proceedings. Pearson and Thoennes found an agreement rate of 60 per cent, which they argue 'falls squarely in the range reported in the literature' (1984:514); the majority of those who experienced the process were pleased with it, regarding it as both fair and just. This view was also partly shared by those who failed to reach agreements, although the long-term outcome of such cases was not so positive.

The evidence for the effectiveness of conciliation in Britain is even more sparse, although favourable claims have been made. There are also various methodological issues to be resolved such as the importance of distinguishing between a settlement, in the sense of the end of the dispute and overt conflict, and a resolution of the issues in the sense of removing the causes of the conflict. Davis (1983) also points to the remarkable consistency of 'success rates' produced by various mediation procedures, suggesting the importance of in-built pressures moving the parties towards settlement, and the need to account for both the timing and the quality of any settlements reached. On the basis of his research into the Bristol Courts Family Conciliation Service (Davis 1982a), he concludes that conciliation does help to resolve disputes and therefore offers a more satisfactory way of dealing with divorce disputes than is available by other means, which may even save money. Until the work of the Conciliation Project Unit proposed by the Inter-departmental Committee on Conciliation (Lord Chancellor's Department 1983) has been completed, however, the argument in Britain over the effectiveness of conciliation is likely to be conducted on the basis of faith rather than fact.

A model of conciliation

The diversity of current practice and the confusion surrounding this has already been referred to. Arising from the foregoing discussion, we would propose the following as a model of practice that might be helpful in pulling together much of this material into a more coherent and practical form.

INTRODUCTORY STAGE

All sessions should be conducted by two conciliators. It may be that a male/female pairing may have some advantages, but such a view would be speculative and may not be practicable. Careful attention should be given to physical matters such as arranging seating non-hierarchically, preferably in a circle without a table, to encourage a feeling of openness, trust, and face-to-face communication, and to such matters as shaking hands to establish contact and full, possibly informal introductions. The considerable importance of these initial arrangements has been referred to by many (Coogler 1978, Folberg and Taylor 1984, Haynes 1981, Scott 1981), since they are the foundations on which the process is built. The nature of the service and the process of conciliation, as well as the principles underlying it, are explained by one of the conciliators, including the expectation that sessions will normally last about one and a half hours, and that up to a normal maximum of about eight sessions will be offered, although a settlement is often achieved in less than this. The role and contribution of the children is discussed as well as confidentiality and the limits of this, which might arise if child-welfare issues cause concern. The legally privileged nature of the discussions[1] is also outlined, as well as agreed procedures for communicating with solicitors if necessary.

The conciliators should also delineate some of the rules that might be negotiated to control the process, all the time seeking confirmation that the procedures are being understood and agreed by both parents, and stressing that it is a process involving the family and therefore no separate discussions will be entered into with either parent. Even agreement about such procedural issues has symbolic importance at this stage in the process and may provide opportunities for the conciliators to reinforce positive attitudes and responses. Each parent should then be asked to indicate what they feel are the main issues for conciliation; these will then form the basis for an agreement, verbal or written, on the focus of conciliation. The conciliators will therefore be concerned to try to clarify and partialize issues as a means of constructing an agenda, which should be headed by the least difficult issues. Coogler (1978) has suggested that, where custody is an issue, it is almost always wise to seek an agreement on access before seeking a decision about custody and care and control. Frequency of meetings can also be discussed.

The objectives at this stage are to establish an appropriate atmosphere that is supportive, optimistic, and therefore conducive to conciliation, and agreement to a structure for the discussions and the process as a whole, including the importance of the children and ways of dealing with issues in their presence. At the end of the session, the matters agreed should be reviewed and summarized, perhaps in writing, and a mutually convenient time for the next meeting arranged, perhaps with each parent being asked to consider possible areas of agreement in the interim.

THE CONCILIATING STAGE

At the second meeting, a conciliator should remind the parents and the children what was agreed at the introductory meeting in terms of the agenda and procedures. The conciliators should decide before meetings who will assume responsibility for initiating the meeting in this way and other relevant issues. Depending upon the ages of the children, seating may need to be rearranged, and toys, or pens and paper, provided. A conciliator should then invite one parent to initiate the discussion by expressing any views or proposals that they might have concerning the first issue to be decided. The other parent should then be invited to respond and the process will be under way, with the conciliators intervening when necessary and using the various techniques described above to ensure that each parent has a fair hearing, and to begin moving towards an agreement. No pressure should be put on the children to participate in the discussion, but every opportunity should be given for them to contribute if they so wish.

Various techniques, such as role-play, sculpting, or genograms, may be used in order to improve communication and the identification and expression of problems. The conciliators must feel free to comment on each other's interventions if necessary, and even to suggest a short withdrawal to discuss problems that may arise; the nature of these discussions should subsequently be shared with the family if an open and trusting atmosphere is to be maintained. At the end of the session, progress should be summarized and any agreements clarified. If work is still going on, the session should not end simply because the agreed time has elapsed, although the conciliators may remind the parents of the agreed time limits. *Flexible* control over the proceedings is the essence of the process of conciliation. It is always helpful to summarize progress, however, to compliment parents on their efforts and progress, and to draw out the agreements rather than the disagreements. It may also be useful at some stages in this part of the process to move towards some short-term goals – e.g. access arrangements for the next two weeks – which will allow the establishment and development of trust if they work, and a clear focus for discussion if they do not. Each subsequent session should continue this process as the parents work through the issues they initially identified, and other members of the family system, such as grandparents or cohabitees, should be invited to attend if they appear to be significant in resolving the problems and might help the parents to agree. Sufficient time must be allowed to identify and work through, either directly or indirectly, the cause of the conflict that is preventing agreement. Failure to do this may simply cause the conflict to shift to another issue.

THE AGREEMENT STAGE

Agreement may be arrived at relatively early on in the process, in which case the firmness of any such agreement might be tested by means of a 'trial period'. Indeed, parents might feel that this would be desirable even if the process has been lengthy. The conciliators should be prepared to consider such requests and to arrange a further meeting to assess progress and sort out any residual problems. The precise terms of any final agreement should be clarified and put in writing for both parents and their legal representatives, if any. Tentative agreements that may have legal implications may be clarified by telephone contact with a solicitor if there is any doubt. It is also important in ending conciliation, whether agreement has been reached fully, partially, or not at all, to 'leave the door open' to the parents to seek further conciliation. Circumstances and needs can change, and the experience of conciliation may have initiated a process of change that subsequently may make an agreement possible even if there is no, or only little, initial success.

Whilst other writers have developed more complex models, some of which involve separate meetings with either parent, the development of a family profile, occasional diversions into therapy, or other features, the model we have outlined above is derived from what we believe to be both the theoretical underpinnings and the overarching principles of conciliation. It does not provide an exhaustive analysis of the many complex processes that can and do occur, but is intended to provide a sufficiently flexible framework to allow for development, which is also based upon clear statements of principle and a recognition of the nature of conciliation as a method, and the context in which it is developing.

The present situation

The increasing concern in recent years with the ever-growing rate of marital breakdown has given rise to a number of responses, both at a self-help level and the organization of various counselling services or divorce experience courses. These are usually provided by statutory social work agencies and in particular by probation services, in response to an awareness of the need that many people feel for some form of help after their marriage has broken down. Such services, whilst valuable, are not conciliation as a distinctive method of dispute settlement, however. Conciliation in this particular sense can be divided into four separate areas, as we have already argued. The development of each of these is likely to be influenced in particular by the report of the Inter-departmental Committee on Conciliation (Lord Chancellor's Department 1983) and the findings and any recommendations of the Conciliation Project Unit recommended therein. The recent proposals (Lord Chancellor's Department 1985) of the committee established in August 1982, under the chairmanship of Mrs Justice Booth, to examine procedures under the Matrimonial Causes Act 1973, and to recommend reforms that might, amongst other things, mitigate the intensity of disputes in divorce and encourage settlements, will also be important. Until this process of research and review is completed, statutory change seems unlikely, and uncertainty will continue.

The other areas, involving 'in-court' conciliation by the probation service – especially following the recommendations of the Booth Committee (Lord Chancellor's Department 1985: para. 3.13) encouraging local initiatives – and out-of-court schemes run by voluntary specialist agencies, seem likely to expand. We would nevertheless argue that much of the work done by individual probation officers in the process of preparing welfare reports, which is often termed 'conciliation', constitutes a conciliatory approach but *not* conciliation as a method as we have defined it. As we have written elsewhere (James and Wilson 1984a), there is much real and potential confusion surrounding this area of practice, both for the officers concerned and for the clients with whom they have contact. Not only could the attempt to conciliate cause confusion when the parties anticipate an investigation prior to the preparation of a report, but such an attempt might also prejudice the officer's impartiality, both real and perceived, in such a situation, raising questions about the justice of such an approach: 'welfare investigation and conciliation have different objectives and are based upon different principles (Davis 1982a:125). Other issues of justice are raised by such an approach, especially where the courts might collude with attempts to conciliate by agreeing to sometimes considerable delays in the eventual hearing whilst the officer seeks agreement. In such a situation, if no agreement is reached the delays involved, together with the courts' tendency to maintain the status quo, may substantially damage a non-custodial parent's claim for custody. Whilst such an approach does have its proponents (e.g. Wilkinson 1981), the confusions and potential dangers are many.

Conciliation, as practised by many civil work teams in the probation service, none the less constitutes a distinct method, although the models of practice used may vary. Indeed, the very scale of such developments means that much important work is being done in such teams to test new approaches and develop new models of practice. The involvement of the probation service and court welfare officers in conciliation raises important issues; 'a strong case can be made for keeping mediatory forms of intervention quite *separate from the places and personnel of the law*' (Roberts 1983:557, emphasis added). Greater proximity to the legal system may well affect the perception of parents being invited to attend for conciliation, and there is a danger that 'The authority of the court will bring greater pressure on the parties and their own emotional resistances will be given less weight' (Davis 1982a:124) the closer that conciliation takes place to the courts. This is certainly an issue to which careful consideration must be given when addressing the question of whether conciliation should form part of the statutory legal process or not. Whilst compulsory conciliation may produce a high level of attendance, it may also result in lower motivation to resolve as opposed to settle issues, and a lower commitment to any settlement reached. There is also some evidence from Europe (Schmidt 1984) that such a system can become routinized and therefore devalued, although it seems to work successfully in some countries.

Of more fundamental importance is the tension existing between conciliation and the present responsibilities that the service has to provide a welfare service for the courts, which includes investigating and reporting upon matters concerning the welfare of children. An issue of practice arises when conciliation is not successful and a welfare report is required. Since discussions in conciliation are privileged, it seems inappropriate for those involved in the conciliation attempt to prepare a welfare report subsequently, a view reflected by the recommendation of the Booth Committee that these functions should be separated (Lord Chancellor's Department 1985: para. 4.63). Indeed, the recognition by the parties that this might happen may well influence the process of conciliation, whilst failure to inform the parties that it might happen should conciliation be unsuccessful raises clear ethical problems.

An issue of principle is also raised by this same tension, in so far as welfare officers undertaking conciliation may have cause to be concerned about the welfare of the children. This is an issue for conciliation as a method, whether practised by statutory or by voluntary agencies, since although conciliation stresses the self-determination of the parents and their responsibility for making decisions concerning the children, conciliators cannot allow themselves to be party to any decision that clearly disadvantages any of the individuals involved, especially the children. This overall moral and ethical constraint is compounded by the general responsibility that court welfare officers have for the welfare of children in divorce proceedings, a responsibility that the service must not lose sight of in its enthusiasm to develop a more constructive approach to divorce. As Davis argues, it is important that the probation service should manage the development of its conciliation work in a way allowing it 'sufficient flexibility to establish clear boundaries between different areas of its civil work' (1982a: 128). It must also recognize that, as Perlman's (1957) problem-solving approach highlights, the place in which the process occurs and the overall function of the agency are important factors, since they can create various pressures and tensions that can have a profound impact on the helping process; the fact the civil work functions of the probation service are now its lowest priority (Home Office 1984) must also be borne in mind.

Voluntary out-of-court schemes are the other major setting for the development of conciliation. Apart from the financial difficulties resulting from the lack of public money, these schemes seem likely to grow. Conciliation through such schemes is likely to be available much earlier in the divorce process; but as Parkinson (1983b) has argued, there is some reason to believe that such schemes might end up catering for primarily middle-class clients. There is also evidence of a much higher rate of attrition amongst referrals compared with in-court schemes, which are vested with greater authority. In addition, although such schemes have the advantage of specialization, there is a proper concern by organizations such as the National Family Conciliation Council about the need to maintain proper ethical, practice, and training standards amongst a large number of schemes, the origins and management of which are diverse and variable in terms of quality. As we have argued elsewhere (James and Wilson 1984b), however, there is a case for the complementarity of in-court and out-of-court services, both of which have their own strengths and weaknesses and both of which have an important contribution to make to the development of conciliation.

Summary

Conciliation, as an aspect of social work with marital problems, is different from the other approaches discussed in this book. It has not emerged from either the theory or practice of social work *per se*, but from a growing recognition of the inadequacy of the approach of the current legal system to settling the problems that arise in many cases out of the breakdown of marriage. An adversarial legal approach may be the only way of resolving some situations, either because of their complexity, or because some spouses may continue to *want* to fight for a settlement and to feel that they have had 'their day in court', a right that the law allows them. Whilst conciliation may not be the best method for all, however, it should be made widely available, since it offers for a great many a considerable improvement as a means of reorganizing family life over the current system, which not only fails to ease conflict, but even exacerbates it. As Visher and Visher poignantly express it, 'Anger and guilt can tie two people together as tightly as love' (1982a: 93), resulting in all the acrimony, conflict, and disruption in the lives of both parents and children so often associated with marital breakdown and divorce. Conciliation aims to resolve such disputes and thereby to cut, or at least to loosen, this particular Gordian knot.

Such an exercise is fully justifiable in its own right. The contribution that social work and other professions can make must be encouraged and explored further because of this. Moreover, as indicated in Chapter 2, at a time when increasing numbers of divorced people remarry, the existence of unresolved problems from former marriages can be a substantial source of stress and conflict for new relationships. Conciliation may therefore also have an important contribution to make to marital stability in many potential and actual step-families. This is not to suggest that conciliation should be conceived of as a service for step-families; rather that, in pursuing the objectives of resolving disputes and conflict, this may be one of the benefits accruing from the development of conciliation.

We have also referred to some of the conceptual and practical confusions surrounding conciliation, drawing attention to some of the sources of these whilst also attempting to clarify them. This is an exercise of fundamental importance, since only from such an exercise can a coherent and integrated approach to conciliation be evolved. It is also an exercise that will continue for some time, in view of the relative newness of both the concept and the awareness of the problems it seeks to ameliorate. An inevitable result of this is that in the meantime, for those in the vanguard of these developments, there will continue to be some confusion and anxiety about the nature and course of developments in the practice of conciliation; Kahn and Earle argue that 'The most difficult task of all is to hold onto the uncertainty while it is still being creative' (1982:15). Paradoxically, this is a task faced not only by those attempting to solve the many problems thrown up by the breakdown of their marriages who seek help through conciliation. It is also faced by all those who would offer help to those experiencing marital problems to whom this book is addressed, but for whom we will still not have been able to provide all the answers to the many questions raised, and for whom a degree of uncertainty will continue.

Note

1   Whilst the extent of legal privilege in out-of-court conciliation has yet to be tested in court, it is widely believed that any such communications would be regarded as privileged. There is no doubt, however, that communications that are part of in-court conciliation would be treated as privileged, unless the parties waived that right.

Appendix: The law relating to marital breakdown in England and Wales

A book about social work with marital problems is written on the assumption that appropriate social-work intervention can often assist couples to avoid the ultimate breakdown of the relationship. The inclusion of a chapter on conciliation, however, also recognizes that such efforts are not always successful and that different forms of helping are more appropriate under such circumstances. One such form of helping may involve giving clients basic information and advice concerning their legal position, and this Appendix is written with that need in mind. It is not intended therefore to provide a detailed analysis of the law relating to marital breakdown, but a concise and non-technical outline of the main grounds for legal action and the major remedies available, which will be relevant in the vast majority of situations. Detailed professional legal advice should always be sought where any doubt exists; but a guiding principle in both domestic and divorce courts is that, where minor children are involved, their welfare shall be the first and paramount consideration in relation to questions regarding custody and upbringing.

Domestic court

Magistrates who have a particular interest or experience in family matters sit in the domestic court. Such courts have traditionally been seen as providing a quicker means of resolving urgent matrimonial issues and as being more accessible than county courts, although as divorce has become more speedy and more readily available, this is now less true.

The domestic court has three main functions, and its principal powers are derived from the Guardianship of Minors Act 1971, the

Domestic Proceedings and Magistrates' Courts Act 1978, and the Magistrates' Courts Act 1980. These main functions are:

(a) *To provide orders relating to maintenance, custody, and access where no divorce action is pending.* Magistrates' matrimonial law now embodies the principle that it is the duty of each spouse to support the other on the basis of equality, although the wife will be the applicant in the majority of cases. Financial provision for a wife (or husband) and children of the family can be made if she can establish *either* that her husband has failed to provide a reasonable level of maintenance for her or the children, *or* that his behaviour is such that she cannot reasonably be expected to live with him, *or* that he has deserted her. The court can also make orders relating to the maintenance of the children, even if the wife (or husband) cannot establish her own entitlement to maintenance under one of these conditions. The conduct of the spouse is no longer relevant to the issue of entitlement to maintenance, however, save in exceptional cases where the court believes that the conduct was such that to disregard it would be inequitable. Orders may include periodical payments, which can be backdated to when the application was made, and a lump sum not exceeding £500 for the applicant and £500 for each child (a figure that may be raised by the Secretary of State) to cover, for example, bills that have fallen due since the separation. Consent orders, where financial arrangements have been agreed by the parties, may also be made. In making any order relating to financial relief, however, the court must now give first consideration to the welfare of any child of the family who has not reached the age of eighteen. In addition, when considering an application for an order for financial provision, the court must also consider whether there is any prospect for reconciliation between the parties, in which case the proceedings may be adjourned.

The domestic court can also make orders vesting the custody of the children in one party, although it need not do so. *Legal* custody may only be given to one person, who will also be given *actual* custody, which means the day-to-day care and control of a child. The court may also order however that a parent who is not given legal custody may retain some or all of the parental rights and duties that comprise legal custody, other than actual custody. Such rights and duties include limited rights relating to education, religion, discipline, and consent to marry. They do not include the right to change a child's name, however. Such an order allows the domestic court in effect to make a form of joint custody order. The parent who is not awarded legal custody will normally be given an order granting reasonable access to the children, and such an order can also be granted to grandparents. The court can also order that children under eighteen should be placed under the supervision of a probation officer or the social services department, or, exceptionally, having heard representations from that department, that they should be made subject to care orders.

(b) *To provide an alternative means of obtaining protection and exclusion orders to applying for an injunction in the county court.* The domestic court can make a protection order if it can be proved that one spouse, usually the husband, has either used or threatened the use of violence against the other or a child of the family, and if the court believes that such an order is necessary to prevent the repetition of such behaviour. In urgent cases, there is the provision for the making of expedited protection orders. In the case of *actual* violence against the wife, children, or a third party, or the contravention of an existing protection order, the court may order the husband to leave the matrimonial home and attach a power of arrest to the protection order. Such orders can be applied for independently of any other proceedings relating to maintenance or custody. A husband who disobeys such an order may be ordered to pay up to £50 for every day he is in default (up to a maximum of £1,000); or the court may commit him to prison for up to two months, although such a committal would normally be suspended.

(c) *To provide both a collection and a payment agency for maintenance orders and a means for varying such orders in response to changes in the parties' circumstances.* The domestic court will normally direct that maintenance be paid to the court collecting officer as opposed to the wife direct. Orders made in the High Court or the county court may also be administered in the same way. The domestic court therefore also has functions relating to the enforcement of such orders. Arrears of maintenance are dealt with by the court, which may, where it decides that failure to pay has been due to wilful refusal or culpable neglect, make an attachment of earnings order directing an employer to deduct the appropriate amount from the husband's earnings, or make a suspended committal order rendering the husband liable to a sentence of up to six weeks in the event of his failure to pay the maintenance ordered and to discharge the arrears as ordered by the court.

Divorce court

As a result of a series of changes in legislation, divorce is now easier to obtain and, in the majority of cases, more speedily obtained than ever before. The main powers of the divorce court are derived from the Matrimonial Causes Act 1973 as amended by the Matrimonial and Family Proceedings Act 1984, the Matrimonial Causes Rules 1977, and the Matrimonial Homes Act 1983. A spouse may not petition for divorce until one year after the date of the marriage, although matters occurring during this period may form the basis of a subsequent petition. Furthermore, the sole ground for divorce is now the irretrievable breakdown of the marriage, which can be established only by proving one or more of the following five facts:

1 that the respondent has committed adultery and the petitioner finds it intolerable to live with the respondent;
2 that the respondent has behaved in such a way that the petitioner cannot reasonably be expected to live with the respondent;
3 that the respondent has deserted the petitioner for a continuous period of at least two years immediately preceding the presentation of the petition;
4 that the parties have lived apart for a continuous period of at least two years immediately preceding the presentation of the petition, and the respondent consents to a decree being granted;
5 that the parties have lived apart for a continuous period of at least five years immediately preceding the presentation of the petition.

The majority of divorce petitions, about 98 per cent, are undefended and are heard in a simplified 'special procedure', which, in most cases, does not require the attendance of the petitioner or witnesses at court. Defended divorce cases are heard in the Family Division of the High Court. The court has the duty to deal with the issue of the dissolution of the marriage and then to deal with the question of 'ancillary relief' — i.e. custody, care and control, and access with regard to the children, and maintenance and property issues. Even though some of these issues are not infrequently contested, they are still dealt with in the county court where the divorce petition itself is undefended.

CUSTODY AND ACCESS

Before a decree can be made absolute, the court must have determined who are the children of the family — i.e. a child of whom both parties are the parents, or any other child (other than a foster-child) who has been treated by both parties as a child of the family. Having considered the arrangements that have been made for their welfare, the court must make a declaration that these are satisfactory or the best that can be devised in the circumstances. This process applies to every child under the age of 16, any child under 18 who is receiving vocational or educational training, and any child over 18 to whom the court considers it should apply for special reasons such as physical or mental handicap. Delays may occur in compiling sufficient informa- tion to enable the judge to make a declaration of satisfaction, and in such cases, although a decree nisi cannot normally be made absolute until after the 'children's appointment' at which the arrangements are considered, it is possible for this to be done if the parties wish the decree to be made absolute as soon as possible.

Normally, the court will award both *custody* and *care and control* to one parent only, and orders that split these two functions are avoided. Another possibility, which is receiving increasing attention, however, is the *joint* custody order in which both parents share custody, with one parent retaining care and control. Such an order may often be the out- come of conciliation and may be made where it is intended and expected that both parents will be involved co-operatively in bringing up and caring for the children. Such orders also lessen the appearance of there being a winner and a loser, a custodial and a non-custodial parent, and underline the continuing role of both parents after divorce. County courts can also make interim custody orders in cases where there is some urgency, such as soon after the separation where parents can- not agree on who should look after the children, or where the party who is not looking after the children has indicated an intention to contest custody, in which case a full hearing may be delayed until after the divorce. As with the domestic court, a child under the age of eighteen can also be placed under the supervision of a probation officer or the social services department, or, exceptionally, be made the subject of a care order.

Orders relating to access are frequently made pending the resolu- tion of custody disputes. Once the issue of custody has been settled, however, courts will almost invariably make an order for reasonable access, leaving it to the parties to determine the nature and frequency of access. Less frequently, an order defining aspects such as the dates, times, frequency, and duration of access may be made. Since access is often a focus for conflict, such defined access orders are rarely a satis- factory solution, because, although the court does in theory have the power to enforce access by the committal of an obstructive custodial parent to prison for contempt or to transfer custody to the other parent, in practice the enforcement of such orders is virtually impossible.

PROPERTY AND FINANCIAL ARRANGEMENTS

Once the breakdown of the marriage has been established, the court often has to decide which party should live in the matrimonial home. In cases where there are delays in dealing with other issues, or where violence has been threatened or has occurred, action in relation to the matrimonial home may be necessary in advance of other property and financial issues. In such cases, the court has the power to make an 'ouster' injunction, even where the applicant has no legal title to the property. Such proceedings are quite separate from any divorce proceedings even though they may arise out of the same general circumstances. Similarly a non-molestation injunction, which is similar to a protection order made in the domestic court, can be issued and may frequently be considered alongside an application for interim custody or an 'ouster' injunction, although the consequences of such an order for future positive communication between the spouses where there are children involved should be carefully considered. Such an injunction may be made with an added power of arrest for breach, which may be dealt with by the court using its powers in relation to contempt.

The many provisions of the law with regard to property and financial matters are too detailed and complex to be considered here. Indeed, such detailed knowledge is scarcely needed by social workers, and such matters are best left to the legal profession. Certain principles can be made clear, however. In making decisions on financial relief or the matrimonial home, the court must give first consideration to the welfare of any child of the family who has not attained the age of eighteen; and, in this respect, the standard of living enjoyed before the marriage broke down is one of the factors the court may consider. The conduct of the parties is no longer a major issue in determining financial relief and property orders, except in cases where the court feels that the nature of the conduct was such that to disregard it would be inequitable.

Recent changes have seen a move away from the previous provisions, which were felt to encourage long-term dependence on ex-spouses. New provisions emphasize, even in the majority of cases where a clean break financially is not possible, financial support from ex-spouses as being primarily a means of ensuring a smooth transition from marriage to independence and self-sufficiency, subject to the overriding requirement to give first consideration to the welfare of any minor child of the family. Courts now also have the power to make consent orders in relation to financial arrangements based solely on the information contained in the application.

The divorce court also has powers to deal with much rarer matrimonial causes such as nullity and judicial separation, which will not be considered here.

Legal aid

In advising clients in relation to marital breakdown, a social worker may well wish to advise them to consult a solicitor at some stage or in relation to some issues, although conciliation can result in agreement on a range of issues, especially relating to children, on which advice has often been sought from solicitors in the past. Legal advice and assistance are widely available under the Green Form Scheme operated by solicitors who participate in the legal aid scheme. A list of such solicitors who specialize in matrimonial work can be obtained from the local offices of the Law Society. This scheme does not extend to legal representation in court, with the exception of representation in proceedings in the domestic court. Where representation is necessary, a solicitor can apply for a legal aid certificate to the Law Society. Details of such facilities are best obtained from solicitors who participate in the scheme. Legal aid is not available for 'special procedure' divorces, however, because of their simple and straightforward nature, although advice and assistance are available in the normal way through the Green Form Scheme.

Statutory duties

Social workers in probation services and social services departments may also have statutory involvement in the process of marital breakdown. The powers to make supervision and care orders in such proceedings have already been mentioned, but in addition to these, reports can be called for in a variety of situations. In the domestic court, reports can be required to investigate issues concerning custody and access, or means enquiries can be required when considering maintenance orders or arrears in payments. Probation officers can also be requested to explore the possibility of reconciliation between the parties. In the divorce court, a judge or a registrar can refer to a court welfare officer any matter concerning the welfare of a child at any time, and the parties themselves can request the registrar to order such a report. Such reports include pre-decree reports, satisfaction reports, contested custody reports, disputed access reports, and interim custody reports. All such enquiries and reports are for different purposes and will therefore vary in how they are carried out and presented; readers are referred elsewhere for a discussion of the many issues related to this. Such investigatory and report-writing activities are frequently used as an opportunity for conciliation, however, as we have noted above in our discussion of this subject.

The law relating to marital breakdown is not only complex but has, in recent years, been the subject of many changes. Whilst this Appendix was accurate at the time of going to press, therefore, the reader should be alert to the possibility of further changes. The Booth Committee (Lord Chancellor's Department 1985) has recently made its final proposals for the simplification of procedures relating to matrimonial causes. These are substantial and include the introduction of an initial hearing for divorce applications early on in the process, in every case involving children of the family, at which conciliation would be available and consent orders could be made (by a registrar in some circumstances), and where final orders could be made even in contested matters that are relatively straightforward. Other changes are proposed relating to a range of issues including injunctions and urgent applications, ancillary relief, supervision orders, the role and duties of the welfare officer, and the timing of proceedings, all designed to simplify and speed up the process and to facilitate agreed outcomes. In addition, there are likely to be substantial debates about the possible creation of a family court and a continuing debate about the role and development of conciliation, both of which may lead to changes.

Suggestions for further reading

Barnard, D. (1983) *The Family Court in Action*. London: Butterworths.

Consumers Association (1984) *Divorce: Legal Procedures and Financial facts*. London: Consumers Association.

Freeman, M. and Lyon, C. (1980) *The Matrimonial Jurisdiction of Magistrates*. Chichester: Barry Rose.

Hoggett, B. (1981) *Parents and Children* (2nd edn). London: Sweet & Maxwell.

Maidment, S. (1984) *Child Custody and Divorce*. Beckenham: Croom Helm.

Wilkinson, M. (1981) *Children and Divorce*. Oxford: Blackwell.

References

Agazarian, Y. and Peters, R. (1981) *The Visible and Invisible Group: Two Perspectives on Group Psychotherapy and Group Process.* London: Routledge & Kegan Paul.

Ahmed, S. (1981) Asian Girls and Culture Conflict. In J. Cheetham, W. James, M. Loney, B. Mayor, and W. Prescott (eds) *Social and Community Work in a Multi-Racial Society: A Reader.* London: Harper & Row.

—— (1983) Blinkered by Background. *Community Care* 483, 13 October.

Ahrons, C. (1980) Redefining the Divorced Family: a conceptual framework. *Social Work* 25(6).

Albrecht, S. (1979) Correlates of Marital Unhappiness Among the Remarried. *Journal of Marriage and the Family* 41(4).

Ambrose, P., Harper, J., and Pemberton, R. (1983) *Surviving Divorce: Men Beyond Marriage.* Brighton: Wheatsheaf.

Anderson, M. (1972) Household Structure and the Industrial Revolution; mid-nineteenth-century Preston in comparative perspective. In P. Laslett with R. Wall (eds) *Household and Family in Past Time.* Cambridge: Cambridge University Press.

Archer, J. (1982) A Winter's Tale. *British Journal of Social Work* 12(2).

Askham, J. (1984) *Identity and Stability in Marriage.* Cambridge: Cambridge University Press.

Association of Directors of Social Services (1983) *Social Services and Ethnic Minorities: A Report of the Training and Staff Development Sub-Committee.* Newcastle: ADSS.

Atma, R. (1985) The Asian Counselling Service. *Marriage Guidance*, Summer.

Baird, P. (1978) The Evaluation of Social Work Practice. In M. R. Olsen (ed) *The Unitary Model: Its Implications for Social Work Theory and Practice*. Birmingham: British Association of Social Workers.

Ballard, C. (1979) Conflict, Continuity and Change: Second-Generation South Asians. In V. Khan (ed.) *Minority Families in Britain: Support and Stress*. London: Macmillan.

Ballard, R. (1979) Ethnic Minorities and the Social Services: What type of service? In V. Khan (ed.) *Minority Families in Britain: Support and Stress*. London: Macmillan.

—— (1982) South Asian Families. In R. N. Rapoport, M. Fogarty, and R. Rapoport (eds) *Families in Britain*. London: Routledge & Kegan Paul.

Ballard, R. and Ballard, C. (1977) The Sikhs: The Development of South Asian Settlements in Britain. In J. Watson (ed.) *Between Two Cultures: Migrants and Minorities in Britain*. Oxford: Blackwell.

Bannister, K. and Pincus, L. (1965) *Shared Phantasy in Marital Problems*. London: Institute of Marital Studies, Tavistock Institute of Human Relations.

Barbach, L. (1980) Group Treatment of Anorgasmic Women. In S. Leiblum and L. Pervin (eds) *Principles and Practice of Sex Therapy*. London: Tavistock.

Belshaw, C. and Strutt, M. (1984) *Couples in Crisis: Facing Marital Breakdown*. London: Gollancz.

Benedek, R. and Benedek, E (1977) Postdivorce Visitation: A Child's Right. *Journal of the American Academy of Child Psychiatry* 16(2).

Berman, E. and Lief, H. (1975) Marital Therapy from a Psychiatric Perspective: an Overview. *American Journal of Psychiatry* 132(6).

Bernard, S., Folger, J., Weingarten, H., and Zumeta, Z. (1984) The Neutral Mediator: Value Dilemmas in Divorce Mediation. *Mediation Quarterly* 4.

Birchler, G. (1973) Differential Patterns of Instrumental Affiliative Behaviour as a Function of Degree of Marital Distress and Level of Intimacy. In R. Segraves (ed.) (1982) *Marital Therapy*. New York: Plenum.

Birchler, G., Weiss, R., and Vincent, J. (1975) A Multimethod Analysis of Social Reinforcement Exchange between Maritally Distressed and Non-distressed Spouse and Strange Dyads. *Journal of Personality and Social Psychology* 31.

Blades, J. (1984) Mediation: An Old Art Revitalized. *Mediation Quarterly* 3.

Blair, W., Kehra, A., Khoot, S., and Patel, R. (1981) Level Crossing. In J. Cheetham *et al.* (eds) *Social and Community Work in a Multi-Racial Society: A Reader*. London: Harper & Row.

Blood, R. (1965) Long-Range Causes and Consequences of the Employment of Married Women. *Journal of Marriage and the Family* 27(1).

Bott, E. (1971) *Family and Social Network*. London: Tavistock (original edition 1957).

Bottomley, A. (1984) Resolving Family Disputes: a critical view. In M. Freeman (ed.) *The State, The Law and The Family*. London: Tavistock.

Bowerman, C. and Irish, D. (1962) Some Relationships of Stepchildren to their parents. *Marriage and Family Living* 24.

Bowlby, J. (1971) *Attachment*. Harmondsworth: Pelican (original edition 1969).

Bowling, A. (1984) Caring for the Elderly Widowed – the Burden on their Supporters. *British Journal of Social Work* 14(5).

Brannen, J. (1980) Seeking Help for Marital Problems: A Conceptual Approach. *British Journal of Social Work* 10(4).

Brannen, J. and Collard J. (1982) *Marriages in Trouble: The Process of Seeking Help*. London: Tavistock.

Brayshaw, A. (1980) *Public Policy and Family Life*. Discussion Paper No. 3. London: Policy Studies Institute.

British Association of Social Workers (1982) *Social Work in Multi-Cultural Britain*. Birmingham: BASW.

Brown, A. (1979) *Groupwork*. London: Heinemann.

Brown, A. and Kiernan, K. (1981) Cohabitation in Great Britain: evidence from the General Household Survey. *Population Trends* (25), Autumn.

Brown, D. (1982) *The Step-Family: A Growing Challenge for Social Work*. Social Work Monograph No. 4. Norwich: University of East Anglia/SWT.

Brown, G. and Harris, T. (1978) *Social Origins of Depression*. London: Tavistock.

Bull, R. (1984) Social Work and the Marital Relationship. In H. Jones (ed.) *Issues in Social Welfare*. Cardiff: Department of Social Administration, University College.

Bumpass, L. and Sweet, J. (1972) Differentials in Marital Stability. *American Journal of Sociology* 37.

Burbank, F. (1976) The Treatment of Sexual Problems by Group Therapy. In S. Crown (ed.) *Psychosexual Problems*. London: Academic Press.

Burgoyne, J. (1984) *Breaking Even: Divorce, Your Children and You*. Harmondsworth: Penguin.

Burgoyne, J. and Clark, D. (1981) Parenting in Stepfamilies. In R. Chester, P. Diggory, and M. Sutherland (eds) *Changing Patterns of Child-Bearing and Child-Rearing*. London: Academic Press.

—— and —— (1982a) From Father to Stepfather. In M. O'Brien and L. McKee (eds) *The Father Figure*. London: Tavistock.

—— and —— (1982b) Reconstituted Families. In R. N. Rapoport, M. Fogarty, and R. Rapoport (eds) *Families in Britain*. London: Routledge & Kegan Paul.

—— and —— (1984) *Making a Go of It: A Study of Stepfamilies in Sheffield*. London: Routledge & Kegan Paul.

Burke, R. and Weir, T. (1976) Relationship of Wives' Employment Status to Husband, Wife and Pair Satisfaction and Performance. *Journal of Marriage and the Family* 38(2).

Butler, J., Bow, I., and Gibbons, J. (1978) Task-Centred Casework with Marital Problems. *British Journal of Social Work* 8(4).

Camberwell Council on Alcoholism (1980) *Women and Alcohol*. London: Tavistock.

Caplan, G. (1961) *An Approach to Community Mental Health*. London: Tavistock.

Carter, E. and McGoldrick, M. (eds) (1980) *The Family Life Cycle: A Framework for Family Therapy*. New York: Gardner Press.

Central Statistical Office (1979) *Social Trends, 10*. London: HMSO.

—— (1984) *Annual Abstract of Statistics, 120*. London: HMSO.

Cheetham, J. (1981) Open Your Eyes to Strength. *Community Care* 392, 24 December.

Cheetham, J., James, W., Loney, M., Mayor, B., and Prescott, W. (eds) (1981) *Social and Community Work in a Multi-Racial Society: A Reader*. London: Harper & Row.

Chester, R. (1972) Current Incidence and Trends in Marital Breakdown. *Postgraduate Medical Journal* 48.

—— (1980) *A Survey of Recent UK Literature on Marital Problems*. A Report for the Home Office Research Unit (unpublished).

—— (1985a) The Rise of the Neo-Conventional Family. *New Society* 72(1167).

—— (1985b) Marriage in Britain: An Overview of Research. In W.

Dryden (ed.) *Marital Therapies in Britain*, vol. 1. London: Harper & Row.

Chester, R. and Walker, C. (1978) Sexual Experience and Attitudes of British Women. In W. Armytage, R. Chester, and J. Peel (eds) (1980) *Changing Patterns of Sexual Behaviour*. London: Academic Press.

Clegg, H. (1980) Marital Sexual Dysfunction. *Marriage Guidance* 19(4).

Coogler, O. (1978) *Structured Mediation in Divorce Settlement: A Handbook for Marital Mediators*. Lexington: Heath.

Craig, Y. (1974) Marital Crises and the Dying Child. *Marriage Guidance* 15.

Crown, S. (1976) Psychosexual Problems in Marriage. In S. Crown (ed.) *Psychosexual Problems: Psychotherapy, Counselling and Behaviour Modification*. London: Academic Press.

Davis, G. (1982a) Conciliation: A Dilemma for the Divorce Court Welfare Service. *Probation Journal* 29(4).

—— (1982b) Settlement Seeking in Divorce. *New Law Journal* 132.

—— (1983) Conciliation and the Professions. *Family Law* 13.

Davis, G. and Bader, K. (1983) In-Court Mediation Observed – I and II. *New Law Journal*, 15 and 29 April.

Denney, D. (1983) Some Dominant Perspectives in the Literature Relating to Multi-Racial Social Work. *British Journal of Social Work* 13(2).

DHSS (1974) *Report of the Committee on One-Parent Families*. Cmnd 5629. London: HMSO.

Dickes, R. (1984) Interrelationship between Psychoanalysis and Brief Sex Therapy. In C. Nadelson and D. Polonsky (eds) *Marriage and Divorce: A Contemporary Perspective*. London: Guildford Press.

Dicks, H. (1967) *Marital Tensions*. London: Tavistock.

Dominian, J. (1968) *Marital Breakdown*. Harmondsworth: Penguin.

—— (1980) *Marriage in Britain 1945–80*. Occasional Paper No. 1. London: Study Commission on the Family.

Douglas, T. (1979) *Group Processes in Social Work*. London: Wiley.

Dowling, E. (1979) Co-therapy: a clinical researcher's view. In S. Walrond-Skinner (ed.) *Family and Marital Psychotherapy*. London: Routledge & Kegan Paul.

Driver, G. (1982) West Indian Families: an anthropological perspective. In R. N. Rapoport, M. Fogarty, and R. Rapoport (eds) *Families in Britain*. London: Routledge & Kegan Paul.

Duberman, L. (1973) Step-Kin Relationships. *Journal of Marriage and the Family* 35(2).

Dunnell, K. (1979) *Family Formation 1976*. A Survey carried out on behalf of the Population Statistics Division of the Office of Population Censuses and Surveys. London: HMSO.

Duvall, E. (1967) *Family Development*. Philadelphia: Lippincott.

Edwards, G. (1982) *The Treatment of Drinking Problems: A Guide for the Helping Professions*. London: Grant McIntyre.

Eekelaar, J. (1982) Children in Divorce: Some Further Data. *Oxford Journal of Legal Studies* 2(1).

Eekelaar, J. and Clive, E., with Clarke, K. and Raikes, S. (1977) *Custody After Divorce: The Disposition of Custody in Divorce Cases in Great Britain*. Oxford: SSRC Centre for Socio-Legal Studies.

Eekelaar, J. and Maclean, M. (1983) *Children and Divorce: Economic Factors*. Oxford: SSRC Centre for Socio-Legal Studies.

Erikson, E. (1965) *Childhood and Society*. Harmondsworth: Penguin.

Eversley, D. and Bonnerjea, L. (1982) Social Change and Indicators of Diversity. In R. N. Rapoport, M. Fogarty, and R. Rapoport (eds) *Families in Britain*. London: Routledge & Kegan Paul.

Fagin, L. and Little, M. (1984) *The Forsaken Families: The Effects of Unemployment on Family Life*. Harmondsworth: Penguin.

Fairbairn, W. (1954) *Object-Relations Theory of the Personality*. New York: Basic Books.

Ferri, E. (1984) *Stepchildren: A National Study*. A Report from the National Child Development Study. Windsor: NFER/Nelson.

Figley, C. (1973) Child Density and the Marital Relationship. *Journal of Marriage and the Family* 35(2).

Fischer, J. (1978) *Effective Casework Practice: An Eclectic Approach*. London: McGraw-Hill.

Fitzgerald, R. (1973) *Conjoint Marital Therapy*. New York: Aronson.

Fogarty, M., Rapoport, R., and Rapoport, R. N. (1971) *Sex, Career and Family*. London: Allen & Unwin.

Folberg, J. and Taylor, A. (1984) *Mediation: A Comprehensive Guide to Resolving Conflicts without Litigation*. San Francisco: Jossey-Bass.

Foner, N. (1977) The Jamaicans: Cultural and Social Change among Migrants in Britain. In J. Watson (ed.) *Between Two Cultures: Migrants and Minorities in Britain*. Oxford: Blackwell.

Forster, J. (1982) *Divorce Conciliation*. A Study of services in England and abroad with implications for Scotland. Edinburgh: Scottish Council for Single Parents.

Francis, W. (1984a) Out of the Textbooks and into the Consulting Room. *Community Care* 535, 25 October.

—— (1984b) Childlessness: The Hidden Heartache. *Community Care* 536, 1 November.

Freeman, M. (1984) Questioning the Delegalization Movement in Family Law: Do We Really Want a Family Court? In J. Eekelaar and S. Katz (eds) *The Resolution of Family Conflict: Comparative Legal Perspectives*. Toronto: Butterworths.

Furstenberg, F. and Spanier, G. (1984) *Recycling the Family: Remarriage After Divorce*. Beverly Hills: Sage.

Gathorne-Hardy, J. (1981) *Love, Sex, Marriage and Divorce*. London: Cape.

George, V. and Wilding, P. (1972) *Motherless Families*. London: Routledge & Kegan Paul.

Getz, W., Wiesen, A., Sue, S., and Ayers, A. (1974) *Fundamentals of Crisis Counselling*. Lexington: Heath.

Gibbons, J., Bow, I., Butler, J., and Powell, J. (1979) Clients' Reactions to Task-Centred Casework: a Follow-Up Study. *British Journal of Social Work* 9(2).

Gillespie, D. (1971) Who Has the Power? The Marital Struggle. *Journal of Marriage and the Family* 33(3).

Glenn, N. and McLanahan, S. (1982) Children and Marital Happiness: A Further Specification of the Relationship. *Journal of Marriage and the Family* 44(1).

Glenn, N. and Weaver, C. (1977) The Marital Happiness of Remarried Divorced Persons. *Journal of Marriage and the Family* 39(2).

—— and —— (1978) A Multivariate, Multisurvey Study of Marital Happiness. *Journal of Marriage and the Family* 40(2).

Goode, W. (1964) *The Family*. New Jersey: Prentice-Hall.

Goody, E. and Groothues, C. (1977) The West Africans: The Quest for Education. In J. Watson (ed.) *Between Two Cultures: Migrants and Minorities in Britain*. Oxford: Blackwell.

—— and —— (1979) Stress in Marriage: West African Couples in London. In V. Khan (ed.) *Minority Families in Britain: Support and Stress*. London: Macmillan.

Goody, J. (1972) The Evolution of the Family. In P. Laslett with R. Wall (eds) *Household and Family in Past Time*. Cambridge: Cambridge University Press.

Gorer, G. (1971) *Sex and Marriage in England Today: A study of the views and experience of the under-45s*. London: Nelson.

Gorrell Barnes, G. (1984a) *Working with Families*. London: Macmillan/BASW.

—— (1984b) Systems Theories and Family Theories. In M. Rutter and

L. Hersor (eds) *Child Psychiatry: Modern Approaches*. Oxford: Blackwell Scientific Publications.

Gottman, J., Notarius, C., Markman, H., Bank, S., Yoppi, B., and Rubin, M. (1976) Behaviour Exchange Theory and Marital Decision-making. *Journal of Personality and Social Psychology* 34.

Grant, M. and Gwinner, P. (eds) (1979) *Alcoholism in Perspective*. London: Croom Helm.

Greenspan, S. and Mannino, F. (1974) A Model for Brief Interventions with Couples based on Projective Identification. *American Journal of Psychiatry* 131.

Guise, J. (1983) Conciliation: Current Practice and Future Implications for the Probation Service. *Probation Journal* 30(2).

Gullick, E. (1983) The Marital Relationship: Adapting an Old Model to Contemporary Needs. In C. Nadelson and D. Marcotte (eds) *Treatment Interventions in Human Sexuality*. New York: Plenum.

Gulliver, P. (1979) *Disputes and Negotiations: A Cross-Cultural Perspective*. New York: Academic Press.

Gurman, A. (1975a) Evaluating the Outcomes of Couples Groups. In A. Gurman and D. Rice (eds) (1975) *Couples in Conflict*. New York: Aronson.

—— (1975b) Some Therapeutic Implications of Marital Therapy Research. In A. Gurman and D. Rice (eds) (1975) *Couples in Conflict*. New York: Aronson.

—— (1978) Contemporary Marital Therapies: A Critique and Comparative Analysis of Psychoanalytic, Behavioural and Systems Theory Approaches. In T. Paolino and B. McCrady (eds) *Marriage and Marital Therapy*. New York: Brunner/Mazel.

Gurman, A. and Kniskern, D. (1978) Research on Marital and Family Therapy: Progress, Perspective and Prospect. In S. Garfield and A. Bergin (eds) *Handbook of Psychotherapy and Behaviour Change* (2nd edn). Chichester: Wiley.

Gurman, A. and Rice, D. (1975) *Couples in Conflict: New Directions in Marital Therapy*. New York: Aronson.

Guthrie, L. and Mattinson, J. (1971) *Brief Casework with a Marital Problem*. London: Institute of Marital Studies, Tavistock.

Haley, J. (1963) *Strategies of Psychotherapy*. New York: Grune & Stratton.

—— (1971) Family Therapy. *International Journal of Psychiatry* 9.

—— (1976) *Problem-Solving Therapy*. San Francisco: Jossey-Bass.

Hamblin, A. (1970) The World of the Fair: Casework with a

Schizophrenic Patient and his Wife. In Family Welfare Association, *The Voice of Social Work*. Bookstall Services.

Harris, T. (1973) *I'm OK, You're OK*. New York: Cape.

Hart, N. (1976) *When Marriage Ends: A Study in Status Passage*. London: Tavistock.

Haskey, J. (1982) The Proportion of Marriages Ending in Divorce. *Population Trends* 27.

—— (1983a) Children of Divorcing Couples. *Population Trends* 31.

—— (1983b) Marital Status before Marriage and Age at Marriage: their influence on the chance of divorce. *Population Trends* 32.

—— (1983c) Social Class Patterns of Marriage. *Population Trends* 34.

Hawton, K. (1985) *Sex Therapy: A Practical Guide*. Oxford: Oxford University Press.

Haynes, J. (1981) *Divorce Mediation: A Practical Guide for Therapists and Counselors*. New York: Springer.

—— (1983) The Process of Negotiations. *Mediation Quarterly* 1.

Heap, K. (1977) *Group Theory for Social Workers*. Oxford: Pergamon.

—— (1979) *Process and Action in Work with Groups*. Oxford: Pergamon.

Heisler, J. (1984) Employment, Unemployment and Marriage. In the *National Marriage Guidance Council Annual Report*. Rugby: NMGC.

Hicks, M. and Platt, M. (1970) Marital Happiness and Stability: A Review of Research in the Sixties. *Journal of Marriage and the Family* 32(4).

Hobbs, D. and Cole, S. (1976) Transition to Parenthood: A Decade Replication. *Journal of Marriage and the Family* 38(4).

Homans, G. (1961) *Social Behaviour: Its Elementary Forms*. London: Routledge & Kegan Paul.

Home Office (1979) *Marriage Matters: A Working Party Report*. London: HMSO.

—— (1984) Statement of National Objectives and Priorities for the Probation Service in England and Wales.

Hooper, D., Hinchcliff, M., and Roberts F. (1978) *The Melancholy Marriage: Depression in Marriage and Psychosocial Approaches to Therapy*. Chichester: Wiley.

Houseknecht, S. (1979) Childlessness and Marital Adjustment. *Journal of Marriage and the Family* 41(2).

Howard, J. and Shepherd, G. (1982) Conciliation – New Beginnings? *Probation Journal* 29(3).

Humphrey, M. (1975) The Effect of Children upon the Marriage Relationship. *British Journal of Medical Psychology* 48.

Hunt, L. (1982) *Alcohol Related Problems*. London: Heinemann.

Ineichen, B. (1977) Youthful Marriage: The Vortex of Disadvantage. In R. Chester and J. Peel (eds) *Equalities and Inequalities in Family Life*. London: Academic Press.

Jackson, D. (1977) The Study of the Family. In P. Watzlawick and J. Weakland (eds) *The Interactional View*. New York: Norton.

Jackson, D. and Weakland, J. (1971) Conjoint Family Therapy: Some Consideration on Theory, Technique and Results. In J. Haley (ed.) *Changing Families*. New York: Grune & Stratton.

Jacobson, G. (1983) *The Multiple Crisis of Marital Separation and Divorce*. New York: Grune & Stratton.

Jacobson, N. and Margolin, G. (1979) *Marital Therapy*. New York: Brunner/Mazel.

James, A. and Wilson, K. (1984a) Reports for the Court: The Work of the Divorce Court Welfare Officer. *Journal of Social Welfare Law*, March.

—— and —— (1984b) Conciliation – The Way Ahead. *Family Law* 14.

—— and —— (1984c) The Trouble with Access: A Study of Divorcing Families. *British Journal of Social Work* 14(5).

—— and —— (1984d) Towards a Natural History of Access Arrangements in Broken Marriages. In J. Eekelaar and S. Katz (eds) *The Resolution of Family Conflict: Comparative Legal Perspectives*. Toronto: Butterworths.

Jayratne, S. and Levy, R. (1979) *Empirical Clinical Practice*. New York: Columbia University Press.

Jehu, D. (1979) *Sexual Dysfunction: A Behavioural Approach to Causation, Assessment and Treatment*. Chichester: Wiley.

Johnson, H. (1980) Working with Stepfamilies: Principles of Practice. *Social Work* 25(4).

Jung, C. (1925) Marriage as a Psychological Relationship. In *The Development of Personality*, vol. CVII (collected works). London: Routledge & Kegan Paul.

Kahn, J. and Earle, E. (1982) *The Cry for Help and the Professional Response*. Oxford: Pergamon.

Kay, G. (1972) *The Family in Transition*. Newton Abbot: David & Charles.

Keily, G. (1984) Social Change and Marital Problems: Implications for Marriage Counselling. *British Journal of Guidance and Counselling* 12(1).

Kelly, G. (1955) *The Psychology of Personal Constructs: a theory of personality*. New York: Norton.

Kelly, J. (1983) Mediaton and Psychotherapy: Distinguishing the Differences. *Mediation Quarterly* 1.

Kelly, J. and Wallerstein, J. (1977) Part-time Parent, Part-time Child: Visiting after Divorce. *Journal of Clinical Child Psychology* 6.

Kew, S. (1974) Handicap and the Marital Crisis. *Marriage Guidance* 15.

Khan, V. (1977) The Pakistanis: Mirpuri Villagers at Home and in Bradford. In J. Watson (ed.) *Between Two Cultures: Migrants and Minorities in Britain*. Oxford: Blackwell.

—— (ed.) (1979) *Minority Families in Britain: Support and Stress*. London: Macmillan.

Kilmann, P. and Mills, K. (1983) *All About Sex Therapy*. New York: Plenum.

King, K., McIntyre, J., and Axelson, L. (1968) Adolescents' Views of Maternal Employment as a Threat to the Marital Relationship. *Journal of Marriage and the Family* 30(4).

Kinnon, U. (1984) Culture Shock. *Social Work Today* 15(20).

Kitchen, F. (1942) *Brother to the Ox*. London: British Publishers Guild.

Klemer, R. (1970) *Marriage and Family Relationships*. New York: Harper & Row.

Krasner, N., Madden, J., and Walker, R. (1984) *Alcohol Related Problems: Room for Manoeuvre*. Chichester: Wiley.

Lago, C. (1981) Cross-Cultural Counselling: Some Developments, Thoughts and Hypotheses. *New Community* 9(1).

Laslett, P. (1972a) The History of the Family. In P. Laslett and R. Wall (eds) *Household and Family in Past Time*. Cambridge: Cambridge University Press.

—— (1972b) Mean Household Size in England Since the Sixteenth Century. In P. Laslett and R. Wall (eds) *Household and Family in Past Time*. Cambridge: Cambridge University Press.

Lederer, W. and Jackson, D. (1968) *The Mirages of Marriage*. New York: Norton.

Leete, R. (1976) Changing Patterns of Marriage and Remarriage. In R. Chester, and J. Peel (eds) *Equalities and Inequalities in Family Life*. London: Academic Press.

—— (1979) *Changing Patterns of Family Formation and Dissolution* in England and Wales 1964–1976. Studies in Medical and Population Subjects No. 39, Office of Population Censuses and Surveys. London: HMSO.

Leiblum, S. and Pervin, L. (eds) (1980) *Principles and Practice of Sex Therapy*. London: Tavistock.

Lerner, R. and Spanier, G. (eds) (1978) *Child Influences on Marital and Family Interaction: A Life-Span Perspective*. New York: Academic Press.

Levinger, G. (1965) Marital Cohesiveness and Dissolution: An Integrative Review. *Journal of Marriage and the Family* 27(1).

—— (1976) A Social Psychological Perspective on Marital Dissolution. *Journal of Social Issues* 32(1).

Liberman, R. (1975) Behavioural Principles in Family and Couple Therapy. In A. Gurman and D. Rice (eds) (1975) *Couples in Conflict*. New York: Aronson.

—— (1980) *Handbook of Marital Therapy*. New York: Plenum.

Locksley, A. (1980) On the Effects of Wives' Employment on Marital Adjustment and Companionship. *Journal of Marriage and the Family* 42(2).

Lord Chancellor's Department (1983) *Report of the Inter-departmental Committee on Conciliation*. London: HMSO.

—— (1985) *Report of the Matrimonial Causes Procedure Committee*. London: HMSO.

McMasters, E. (1957) Parenthood as Crisis. *Marriage and Family Living* 14(4).

Madge, J. and Brown, C. (1981) *First Homes: A Survey of the Housing Circumstances of Young Married Couples*. London: Policy Studies Institute.

Mainprice, J. (1974) *Marital Interaction and Some Illnesses in Children*. London: Institute of Marital Studies, Tavistock.

Mansfield, P. (1982) A Portrait of Contemporary Marriage: Equal Partners or Just Good Companions. In *Change and Marriage*. Rugby: National Marriage Guidance Council.

Marett, V. (1981) Cross-Cultural Counselling: An Overview of Research. *New Community* 9(1).

—— (1983) *The Resettlement of Ugandan Asians in Leicester: 1972–1980*. Unpublished Ph. D Thesis, University of Leicester.

Marsden, D. (1973) *Mothers Alone*. Harmondsworth: Penguin.

Masters, W. and Johnson, V. (1966) *Human Sexual Response*. London: Churchill.

—— and —— (1970) *Human Sexual Inadequacy*, London: Churchill.

Mattinson, J. and Sinclair, I. (1979) *Mate and Stalemate: Working with Marital Problems in a Social Services Department*. Oxford: Blackwell.

Meissner, W. (1978) The Conceptualisation of Marriage and Family Dynamics from a Psychoanalytic Perspective. In T. Paolino and B. McCrady (eds) *Marriage and Marital Therapy*. New York: Brunner/Mazel.

Messinger, L. (1976) Remarriage between Divorced People with Children from Previous Marriages: A Proposal for Preparation for Remarriage. *Journal of Marriage and Family Counselling* 2.

Miller, B. (1976) A Multivariate Developmental Model of Marital Satisfaction. *Journal of Marriage and the Family* 38(3).

Miller, K. (1963) The Concept of Crisis: Current Status and Mental Health Implications. *Human Organisation* 22.

Minuchin, S. (1974) *Families and Family Therapy*. London: Tavistock.

Mitchell, K. (1984) Work with Ethnic Minorities. *The National Marriage Guidance Council Annual Report*. Rugby: NMGC.

Mnookin, R. and Kornhauser, L. (1979) Bargaining in the Shadow of the Law: The Case of Divorce. *Yale Law Journal* 88.

Morley, R. (1982) Separate but Together – the essential dichotomy of marriage. In *Change and Marriage*. Rugby: National Marriage Guidance Council.

Morris, L. (1985) Responses to Redundancy: Labour-Market Experience, Domestic Organisation and Male Social Networks. *International Journal of Social Economics* 12(2).

Moss, P. and Fonda, N. (1980) *Work and the Family*. London: Temple Smith.

Mount, F. (1982) *The Subversive Family: An Alternative History of Love and Marriage*. London: Cape.

Mueller, C. and Pope, H (1977) Marital Instability: A Study of its transmission between generations. *Journal of Marriage and the Family* 39(1).

Murch, M. (1980) *Justice and Welfare in Divorce*. London: Sweet & Maxwell.

Murdoch, I. (1974) *The Sacred and Profane Love Machine*. London: Chatto & Windus.

Murgatroyd, S. and Woolfe, R. (1982) *Coping with Crisis: Understanding and Helping People in Need*. London: Harper & Row.

Nadelson, C. (1983) Problems in Sexual Functioning. In C. Nadelson and D. Marcotte (eds) *Treatment Interventions in Human Sexuality*. New York: Plenum.

Nissel, M. (1982) Families and Social Change since the Second World War. In R. N. Rapoport, M. Fogarty, and R. Rapoport (eds) *Families in Britain*. London: Routledge & Kegan Paul.

Noller, P. (1984) *Nonverbal Communication and Marital Interaction*. Oxford: Pergamon.

Oakley, A. (1982) Conventional Families. In R. N. Rapoport, M. Fogarty, and R. Rapoport (eds) *Families in Britain*. London: Routledge & Kegan Paul.

Oakley, R. (1982) Cypriot Families. In R. N. Rapoport, M. Fogarty, and R. Rapoport (eds) *Families in Britain*. London: Routledge & Kegan Paul.

Orford, J. and Harwin, J. (eds) (1982) *Alcohol and the Family*. London: Croom Helm.

Osborn, A., Butler, N., and Morris, A. (eds) (1984) *The Social Life of Britain's Five-year-olds*. London: Routledge & Kegan Paul.

Palazolli, M., Boscolo, L., Cecchin, G., and Prata, G. (1978) *Paradox and Counter Paradox: A New Model in the Therapy of the Family in Schizophrenic Transaction*. New York: Aronson.

Parkinson, L. (1983a) Conciliation: A New Approach to Family Conflict Resolution. *British Journal of Social Work* 13(1).

—— (1983b) Conciliation: Pros and Cons (I and II). *Family Law* 13.

—— (1985a) Conciliation in Separation and Divorce. In W. Dryden (ed.) *Marital Therapies in Britain*, vol. II. London: Harper & Row.

—— (1985b) Divorce Counselling. In W. Dryden (ed.) *Marital Therapies in Britain*, vol. II. London: Harper & Row.

Parry, M. (1983) Step-parenthood. *Cambrian Law Review* 14.

Patrician, M. (1984) Child Custody Terms: Potential Contributors to Custody Dissatisfaction and Conflict. *Mediation Quarterly* 3.

Patterson, C. (1978) Cross-Cultural or Inter-Cultural Counselling or Psychotherapy. *International Journal for the Advancement of Counselling* 1(13).

Pearson, G. (1983) *Hooligan: A History of Respectable Fears*. London: Macmillan.

Pearson, J. and Thoennes, N. (1984) Mediating and Litigating Custody Disputes: A Longitudinal Evaluation. *Family Law Quarterly* 17(4).

Perlman, H. (1957) *Social Casework: A Problem Solving Process*. Chicago: University of Chicago Press.

Pill, C. (1981) A Family Life Education Group for Working with Step-parents. *Social Casework* 62(3).

Pincus, A. and Minahan, A. (1973) *Social Work Practice: Model and Method*. Itasca, Ill.: Peacock.

—— and —— (1977) A Model for Social Work Practice. In H. Specht and A. Vickery (eds) *Integrating Social Work Methods*. London: Allen & Unwin.

Pincus, L. (1960) *Marriage: Studies in Emotional Conflict and Growth*. London: Institute of Marital Studies, Tavistock.

Pincus, L. and Dare, C. (1978) *Secrets in the Family*. London: Faber.

Pitt, B. (1976) Sexual Behaviour in the Elderly. In S. Crown (ed.) *Psychosexual Problems: Psychotherapy, Counselling and Behaviour Modification*. London: Academic Press.

Podolsky, E. (1955) The Emotional Problems of the Stepchild. *Mental Hygiene* 39.

Polonsky, D. and Nadelson, C. (1984) Marital Discord and the Wish for Sex Therapy. In C. Nadelson and D. Polonsky (eds) *Marriage and Divorce: A Contemporary Perspective*. London: Guildford Press.

Rack, P. (1979) Diagnosing Mental Illness: Asians and the psychiatric services. In V. Khan (ed.) *Minority Families in Britain: Support and Stress*. London: Macmillan.

Ransom, J., Schlesinger, S., and Derdeyn, A. (1979) A Stepfamily in Formation. *American Journal of Orthopsychiatry* 49(1).

Rapaport, A. (1974) Mathematics and Cybernetics. In S. Arieti (ed.) *American Handbook of Psychiatry*, vol. 1 (2nd edn). New York: Basic Books.

Rapoport, L. (1970) Crisis Intervention as a Mode of Brief Treatment. In R. Roberts and R. Nee (eds) *Theories of Social Casework*. Chicago: University of Chicago Press.

Rapoport, R. (1963) Normal Crises, Family Structure and Mental Health. *Family Process* 2(1).

—— (1981) *Unemployment and the Family*. London: Family Welfare Association.

Rapoport, R. and Rapoport, R. N. (1976) *Dual-Career Families Re-examined*. London: Martin Robertson.

Rapoport, R., Rapoport, R. N., Strelitz, Z. with Kew, S. (1977) *Fathers, Mothers and Others*. London: Routledge & Kegan Paul.

Rapoport, R. N. and Rapoport, R. (1982) British Families in Transition. In R. N. Rapoport, M. Fogarty, and R. Rapoport (eds) *Families in Britain*. London: Routledge & Kegan Paul.

Reid, W. (1975) A Test of a Task-Centred Approach. *Social Work* 20(1).

Reid, W. and Epstein, J. (1972) *Task Centred Casework*. New York: Columbia University Press..

Reid, W. and Hanrahan, P. (1981) The Effectiveness of Social Work: recent evidence. In E. Goldberg and N. Connelly (eds) *Evaluative Research in Social Care*. London: Heinemann.

Renne, K. (1971) Health and Marital Experience in an Urban Population. *Journal of Marriage and the Family* 33(2).

Rice, D., Fey, W., and Kepecs, J. (1972) Therapist Experience and 'Style' as Factors in Co-therapy. *Family Process* 11(1).

Richards, M. and Dyson, M. (1982) *Separation, Divorce and the Development of Children: A Review*. Cambridge: Child Care and Development Group, University of Cambridge.

Rimmer, L. (1981) *Families in Focus: Marriage, Divorce and Family Patterns*. Occasional Paper No. 6. London: Study Commission on the Family.

Rimmer, L. and Popay, J. (1982) *Employment Trends and the Family*. Occasional Paper No. 10. London: Study Commission on the Family.

Roberts, R. and Nee, R. (eds) (1970) *Theories of Social Casework*. Chicago: University of Chicago Press.

Roberts, S. (1983) Mediation in Family Disputes. *Modern Law Review* 46(5).

Robinson, M. (1980) Stepfamlies: A Reconstituted Family System. *Journal of Family Therapy* 2.

Rollins, B. and Cannon, K. (1974) Marital Satisfaction over the Family Life Cycle: A Reevaluation. *Journal of Marriage and the Family* 36(2).

Rosanova, M. (1983) Mediation: Professional Dynamics. *Mediation Quarterly* 1.

Rosenberg, C. (ed.) (1975) *The Family in History*. Pennsylvania: University of Pennsylvania Press.

Rossiter, C. (1980) *Women, Work and the Family*. A Report of a Survey of *Townswomen* Readers. London: Study Commission on the Family.

Royal College of Psychiatrists (1979) *Alcohol and Alcoholism*. The Report of a Special Committee of the Royal College of Psychiatrists. London: Tavistock.

Runnymede Trust and the Radical Statistics Race Group (1980) *Britain's Black Population*. London: Heinemann.

Rutter, M. (1975) *Helping Troubled Children*. Harmondsworth: Penguin.

—— (1977) *Child Psychiatry: Modern Approaches*. Oxford: Blackwell.

—— (1981) *Maternal Deprivation Reassessed* (2nd edn). Harmondsworth: Penguin.

Rutter, M. and Giller, H. (1983) *Juvenile Delinquency: Trends and Perspectives*. Harmondsworth: Penguin.

Ryder, R. (1973) Longitudinal Data Relating Marital Satisfaction and Having a Child. *Journal of Marriage and the Family* 35(4).

Safilios-Rothschild, C. (1970) The Study of Family Power Structure: A Review 1960–1970. *Journal of Marriage and the Family* 32(4).

Sainsbury, E. (1975) *Social Work with Families*. London: Routledge & Kegan Paul.

Sander, F. (1984) Towards a Functional Analysis of Family Process. In J. Eekelaar and S. Katz (eds) *The Resolution of Family Conflict: Comparative Legal Perspectives*. Toronto: Butterworths.

Saposnek, D. (1983) *Mediating Child Custody Disputes*. London: Jossey-Bass.

Satir, V. (1967) *Conjoint Family Therapy*. Palo Alto: Science & Behavioral Books.

Schaffer, H. (1971) *The Growth of Sociability*. Harmondsworth: Penguin.

Scherz, F. (1970) Theory and Practice of Family Therapy. In R. Roberts and R. Nee (eds) *Theories of Social Casework*. Chicago: University of Chicago Press.

Schmidt, T. (1984) The Scandinavian Law of Procedure in Matrimonial Causes. In J. Eekelaar and S. Katz (eds) *The Resolution of Family Conflict: Comparative Legal Perspectives*. Toronto: Butterworths.

Schulman, G. (1972) Myths that Intrude on the Adaptation of the Stepfamily. *Social Casework* 53(3).

Scott, B. (1981) *The Skills of Negotiating*. Aldershot: Gower.

Scott, J. and Tilly, L. (1975) Women's Work and the Family in Nineteenth-century Europe. In C. Rosenberg (ed.) *The Family in History*. Pennsylvania: University of Pennsylvania Press.

Segal, L. (ed.) (1983) *What Is to Be Done about the Family?* Harmondsworth: Penguin.

Segraves, R. (1978) Conjoint Marital Therapy: a cognitive behavioural model. *Archives of General Psychiatry* 35.

—— (1982) *Marital Therapy*. New York: Plenum.

Sharpe, S. (1984) *Double Identity: The Lives of Working Mothers.* Harmondsworth: Penguin.

Sheldon, B. (1982) *Behaviour Modification.* London: Tavistock.

—— (1983) The Use of Single Case Experimental Designs in the Evaluation of Social Work. *British Journal of Social Work* 13(5).

Shorter, E. (1976) *The Making of the Modern Family.* London: Collins.

Singh, R. (1980) *The Sikh Community in Bradford* (2nd edn). Bradford: Faculty of Community Studies, Bradford College..

Skynner, R. (1976) *One Flesh, Separate Persons.* London: Constable.

Smee, C. and Stern, J. (1978) *The Unemployed in a Period of High Unemployment: Characteristics and Benefit Status.* Government Economic Service Working Paper No. 11. London: HMSO. Quoted in L. Rimmer and J. Popay (1982) *Employment Trends and the Family.* London: Study Commission on the Family.

Smelser, N. (1982) The Victorian Family. In R. N. Rapoport, M. Fogarty, and R. Rapoport (eds) *Families in Britain.* London: Routledge & Kegan Paul.

Smith, D. (1976) *The Facts of Racial Disadvantage: A National Survey,* vol. XLII. Broadsheet No. 560. London: PEP.

—— (1981) *Unemployment and Racial Minorities.* London: Policy Studies Institute.

Spanier, G. and Furstenberg, F. (1982) Remarriage After Divorce: A Longitudinal Analysis of Well-being. *Journal of Marriage and the Family* 44(3).

Spanier, G. and Thompson, L. (1984) *Parting: The Aftermath of Separation and Divorce.* Beverly Hills: Sage.

Stone, L. (1977) *The Family, Sex and Marriage: In England 1500–1800.* London: Weidenfeld & Nicolson.

Stuart, R. (1969) Operant-Interpersonal Treatment for Marital Discord. *Journal of Consulting and Clinical Psychology* 33.

Stuckert, R. (1973) Role Perception and Marital Satisfaction – a configurational approach. In M. Lasswell and T. Lasswell (eds) *Love, Marriage, Family: A Developmental Aproach.* Illinois: Scott, Foresman.

Study Commission on the Family (1980) *Happy Families?* A Discussion Paper on Families in Britain. London: Study Commission on the Family.

Sutton, C. (1979) *Psychology for Social Workers and Counsellors.* London: Routledge & Kegan Paul.

Tebboth, R. (1981) For Better? *Social Work Today* 13(9).

Thibaut, J. and Kelley, M. (1959) *The Social Psychology of Groups*. New York: Wiley.

Thomas, E. (1977) *Marital Communication and Decision Making*. New York: Free Press.

Thomas, E., Walter, C., and O'Flaherty, K. (1974) A Verbal Problem Checklist for Use in Assessing Family Verbal Behaviour. *Behavior Therapy* 5.

Thornes, B. and Collard, J. (1979) *Who Divorces?* London: Routledge & Kegan Paul.

Triseliotis, J. (ed) (1972) *Social Work with Coloured Immigrants and their Families*. London: Oxford University Press.

Tunnadine, L. (1970) *Contraception and Sexual Life: A Therapeutic Approach*. London: Tavistock.

Udry, R. (1981) Marital Alternatives and Marital Disruption. *Journal of Marriage and the Family* 43(4).

Visher, E. and Visher, J. (1978a) Common Problems of Stepparents and their Spouses. *American Journal of Orthopsychiatry* 48(2).

—— and —— (1978b) Major Areas of Difficulty for Stepparent Couples. *International Journal of Family Counselling* 6(2).

—— and —— (1979) *Stepfamilies: A Guide to Working with Stepparents and Stepchildren*. New York: Brunner/Mazel.

—— and —— (1982a) *How to Win as a Stepfamily*. New York: Dembner.

—— and —— (1982b) Children in Stepfamilies. *Psychiatric Annals* 12(9).

Von Bertalanffy, L. (1962) General Systems Theory: A Critical Review. *General Systems Yearbook* 8.

Walczak, Y. with Burns, S. (1984) *Divorce: The Child's Point of View*. London: Harper & Row.

Waldron, J., Roth, C., Fair, P., Mann, E., and McDermott, J. (1984) A Therapeutic Mediation Model for Child Custody Dispute Resolution. *Mediation Quarterly* 3.

Walker, C. (1977) Some Variations in Marital Satisfaction. In R. Chester and J. Peel (eds) *Equalities and Inequalities in Family Life*. London: Academic Press.

Walker, L., Brown, H., Crohn, H., Rodstein, E., Zeisel, E., and Sager, C. (1979) An Annotated Bibliography of the Remarried, the Living Together and their Children. *Family Process* 18(2).

Wallerstein, J. and Kelly, J. (1980) *Surviving the Breakup: How Children Cope with Divorce*. London: Grant McIntyre.

Walrond-Skinner, S. (1976) *Family Therapy: The Treatment of Natural Systems*. London: Routledge & Kegan Paul.
—— (ed.) (1979) *Family and Marital Psychotherapy*. London: Routledge & Kegan Paul.
Watson, J. (1984) Appraisal of Marital Problems in the Context of Psychosexual Disturbance. *British Journal of Guidance and Counselling* 12(1).
Watson, J.L. (1977) The Chinese: Hong Kong Villagers in the British Catering Trade. In J. Watson (ed.) *Between Two Cultures*. Oxford: Blackwell.
Watzlawick, P., Beavin, J., and Jackson, D. (1967) *Pragmatics of Human Communication*. New York: Norton.
Watzlawick, P., Weakland, J., and Fisch, R. (1974) *Principles of Problem Formation and Problem Resolution*. New York: Norton.
Weinreich, P. (1979) Ethnicity and Adolescent Identity Conflicts: A Comparative Study. In V. Khan (ed.) *Minority Families in Britain: Support and Stress*. London: Macmillan.
Weiss, R. (1975) *Marital Separation*. New York: Harper & Row.
—— (1978) The Conceptualisation of Marriage from a Behavioural Perspective. In T. Paolino and B. McCrady (eds) *Marriage and Marital Therapy*. New York: Brunner/Mazel.
Weiss, R., Birchler, G., and Vincent, J. (1974) Contractual Models for Negotiation Training in Marital Dyads. *Journal of Marriage and the Family* 36(3).
Weller, R. (1968) The Employment of Wives, Dominance and Fertility. *Journal of Marriage and the Family* 30(3).
West, D. (1982) *Delinquency: Its Roots, Careers and Prospects*. London: Heinemann.
Whitaker, D. (1975) Some Conditions for Effective Work with Groups. *British Journal of Social Work* 5(4).
—— (1976) A Group-Centred Approach. In H. Rabin and M. Rosenbaum (eds) *How to Begin a Psychotherapy Group: Six Approaches*. London: Gordon & Breach.
—— (1985) *Using Groups to Help People*. London: Routledge & Kegan Paul.
Wile, D. (1981) *Couples Therapy*. New York: Wiley.
Wilkinson, M. (1981) *Children and Divorce*. Oxford: Blackwell.
Wise, F. (1977) Conjoint Marital Treatment, In W. Reid and L. Epstein (eds) *Task-Centred Practice*. New York: Columbia University Press.

Wright, J. (1978) Are Working Women Really More Satisfied? Evidence From Several National Surveys. *Journal of Marriage and the Family* 40(2).

Name index

Subject index